TOM NIKKOLA

The 3 Pillars of Vigor

Essential Habits for Exceptional Health and Fitness

First edition

This book was professionally typeset on Reedsy.
Find out more at reedsy.com

Contents

Preface

One sunny Sunday morning during the summer of 2022, my wife Vanessa, our grandson Asher, and I mountain biked through a single-track trail in Woodbury, Minnesota. We knew the trail well. It was one of our favorites. Vanessa always rode in front, then Asher, and then me. That way, we always knew where Asher was, and if either of them fell, I'd be able to help since I rode in the back. We never anticipated the outcome of a ride like the one that Sunday morning.

About halfway through our loop, I rode my bike up a skinny bridge, pedaling slower than I should have. The bridge quickly curved to the right, but my bike went straight. In a split second, my front tire fell from the bridge and hit the ground below. Then, time slowed down. I was almost vertical on my bike as the tire hit the ground, and then I was catapulted from the bike, head-first into the ground. My neck absorbed all that weight, with my body almost completely upside down. Everything went dark, and then at the next moment, I felt my neck snap and saw a flash of light. After that, I lay on my back. My hand throbbed and I had no feeling from the waist down. I knew I'd broken my neck and damaged my spinal cord significantly.

About six months later, I started writing a book. The book wasn't, or isn't, just about recovering from a broken neck. It's about the mental game of life, as well as the importance of being physically prepared for the unexpected. The more I wrote, the more I kept referring to being physically healthy, fit...vigorous. It was as if I was referring to another book I had written. Eventually, I realized I needed to set that book aside and write this one first.

In this book, I take my almost three decades of fitness experience and all the education I've gained along the way and simplify the story about what's necessary to achieve lasting vigor. One of the benefits of achieving such a physical state is that you can bounce back from major injuries much faster, as you'll learn if you read the next book. Beyond recovering from injuries and illness, though, a vigorous body makes you better physically, mentally, professionally, and relationally.

I had a college professor named Dr. Gerald Cizlado at The College of St. Scholastica. He was also my advisor, as I was considering going to medical school after graduation. He was brilliant. And humble. And he made human physiology *so* simple. No matter your knowledge level when you took one of his classes, you could always keep up with his teaching. I learned much from him, but more than anything, I learned to keep things as simple as possible so others can learn and do something with what they learn. I've done my best to keep this book relatively simple while using scientific evidence to support my case in emphasizing The 3 Pillars of Vigor.

I hope it comes across as understandable, relatable, and actionable. The best testimonial I could hope for is a transformational story from you putting these words to action. I hope to see that story one day.

I

Vigor

All vigor is contagious.
– Ralph Waldo Emerson

1

Introduction

The worst part about carrying the milk crate wasn't the weight that made my hands ache, nor was it the relentless taunting from my classmate who strolled behind me, constantly reminding me of my nickname, CP, short for Chubby and Porky. No, the real agony came when the crate's bottom edge would occasionally slam into my shin, sending a jolt of pain that momentarily brought tears to my eyes. Yet, despite the torment, I cherished the responsibility of the "Milk Run." As a third-grader, I would pick up a crate filled with milk cartons from the high school cafeteria and carry the crate to the kindergarten classes, all the while enduring the jibes of the other boy who was supposed to help me carry the crate but usually wouldn't.

I knew the teasing would pass, and completing the milk run was worth it. I knew I was chubby and porky, or as my jeans suggested, "husky." But I had faith that I would someday grow or work my way out of it.

One school day, I recall sitting poolside during swim class, eager for the lesson to begin. As I leaned forward, one of my classmates pointed out my "boobs," larger than most of the girls' in our class. Flushing with embarrassment, I sat back and stretched out my chest, trying to hide the fat hanging from my pecs. I knew that the teasing and my body were temporary.

Today, I am grateful for those difficult moments. They taught me to let go of what others might say about me. They also forced me to confront truths that were not always easy to accept.

Fast-forward eight years, I found myself in the Northern Michigan University cafeteria. On my tray, I lined up four glasses of water and three glasses of diet soda. I placed two slices of turkey and one slice of dry wheat toast on my plate. My breakfast. For lunch, I carried a brown bag that had a sandwich, some vegetables, fruit, and a cookie. I ate the meat from the sandwich and the vegetables. Back at the NMU cafeteria for dinner, I ate a bit of lean protein, a salad with vinegar, and a slice of bread. Of course, I had another four glasses of water and three glasses of diet soda. The water and diet soda helped curb my hunger pangs.

I tried to keep my calories as close to 600 per day as possible, although once per week, I allowed myself a cheat meal, usually on a Friday evening. I'd walk across the street from my dorm to a convenience store. After walking up and down each aisle, salivating at the thought of eating a Snickers bar, a pint of ice cream, or a frozen pizza, I inevitably settled on a loaf of bread and a bottle of salsa. After returning to my dorm room, I ate two salsa sandwiches. Then, I gave the rest of the loaf to someone else or tossed it in the trash.

I was 16 years old and lived on the Northern Michigan University campus with a small group of ski jumpers at the Olympic Training Center, and I took my junior year classes at Marquette High School. Living on the NMU campus, we ate meals in the same cafeteria as the other college students living on campus.

When the school year began, I weighed 157 pounds. At 5'9", I wasn't fat. Not like I had been when I was a pre-teen. But I was still too heavy to be a competitive ski jumper. My coach pulled me aside early in the school year to reinforce this reality. He said, "Tom, if you're going to be serious about the sport, you need to lose weight. You're just too heavy for your height." He was right. At 5'9", 157 pounds was too heavy. If all else is the same about two ski jumpers, the lighter one flies further.

Back then, I often heard that anorexia was more common in ski jumping than in any other Olympic sport, including gymnastics. It got so bad that the International Ski Federation was forced to establish weight minimums for any given skier's height. If they weighed less, they'd be penalized by having to use shorter skis. Since the skis act as wings in flight, this would be a significant handicap for a jumper.

By the time the ski jumping season began that winter, I'd dropped to 137 pounds. I had to cinch my 28" waist jeans with a belt to keep them from falling off. Somehow, while eating only 600 calories and training for two to three hours a day, which often involved miles of running, plyometrics, sprints, and gymnastics if we weren't ski jumping, I maintained a GPA of around 3.8. Thinking back on it today, I understand why my mom was mortified the first time she saw my emaciated face at one of the ski jumping tournaments.

Although I achieved significant weight loss and maintained good grades, my ski jumping career proved inconsistent. By the end of the season, I had accepted that my dream of becoming a world-class ski jumper would never materialize. But this realization led me to a turning point.

I decided to try something new for my workouts. NMU had a very nice gym, and up to that point, I'd never used the weight room out of fear of gaining weight. Since I wasn't worried about that anymore, I took a workout program from a Muscle & Fitness magazine and went to the gym.

The first day I walked into the weight room, I probably looked like a meth addict, but within weeks, I saw my body transform. Lines appeared on my shoulders, my midsection firmed up, and my legs gained strength. I was hooked on this invigorating approach to fitness, and it would guide me for years to come, shaping my life and career.

Three decades later, I have amassed extensive health and fitness experience, getting a pre-med biology degree, working with countless clients, and earning numerous certifications. I spent most of my career working for one of the most respected fitness companies in the U.S., starting out as a personal trainer in 2001 and eventually resigning as a vice president fourteen years later. I also worked for one of the most cutting-edge supplement brands briefly. Today, my wife, Vanessa, and I own and operate various health and fitness-related businesses.

First, I was a fat kid. Then, I was an anorexic teen. But had I not experienced those first two periods in life, I might not have found my way to a gym, where I first discovered the transformative power of strength training. That eye-opening experience ignited a lifelong passion for fitness that has persisted to this day.

From my years of knowledge and practice, I have distilled the most impactful health habits down to what I call The 3 Pillars of Vigor: essential practices that form the foundation of a health-enhancing, fitness-building, and longevity-supporting lifestyle. These three habits play a crucial role in fostering a strong and healthy body and mind. By making them nonnegotiable parts of your life, achieving and maintaining fitness and health will become easier than you ever imagined.

And rest assured, none of the three pillars involve eating salsa sandwiches.

Building Vigor

The term "vigor" has been used throughout history to describe individuals in various ways, often referring to their physical or mental strength, energy, and vitality.

The ancient Greeks used the word "arete" to describe qualities such as courage, excellence, and vigor, which were considered essential for achieving success in diverse fields of life, including warfare, sports, and philosophy.[1] During the Middle Ages, "chivalry" emphasized the importance of vigor and physical prowess in knights and warriors, who were expected to display strength and courage in battle and protect the weak and vulnerable.[2] In the Renaissance, the ideal of the "Renaissance man" highlighted not only physical strength but also intellectual and artistic vigor, as exemplified by figures such as Leonardo da Vinci and Michelangelo.[3]

In the 19th and 20th centuries, "vigor" became increasingly associated with modern ideas of health and fitness. It was during this modern period that people began to emphasize the importance of exercise, nutrition, and other factors in maintaining a strong and healthy body and mind.[4] Today, the word "vigor" is still used to describe individuals who are active, energetic, and vital, whether in the context of sports, business, or personal relationships.[5] It is often seen as a positive attribute associated with strength, resilience, and the ability to overcome challenges and succeed in life.

I'm drawn to the word *vigor* because it encapsulates the

physical state we can all achieve, which unleashes our full potential. Moreover, it is a more traditional word that evokes the values of hard work, embracing challenges, and accepting the truth at face value.

Consider, for example, these words penned by President-elect John F. Kennedy in 1960 in an article he wrote for Sports Illustrated, titled *The Soft American*:

> *Before America becomes great again, it needs to find strength again. Before the country finds strength, its people must attain it first.*
>
> *But the harsh fact of the matter is that there is also an increasingly large number of young Americans who are neglecting their bodies—whose physical fitness is not what it should be—who are getting soft. And such softness on the part of individual citizens can help to strip and destroy the vitality of a nation.*
>
> *For the physical **vigor** of our citizens is one of America's most precious resources. If we waste and neglect this resource, if we allow it to dwindle and grow soft then we will destroy much of our ability to meet the great and vital challenges which confront our people. We will be unable to realize our full potential as a nation.*

Isn't it fascinating how prophetic his words seem today? No doubt, his perspective was shaped by another president sixty years before:

> *In the last analysis a healthy state can exist only when the men and women who make it up lead clean, **vigorous**, healthy lives; when the children are so trained that they*

shall endeavor, not to shirk difficulties, but to overcome them; not to seek ease, but to know how to wrest triumph from toil and risk.
   – President Theodore Roosevelt, The Strenuous Life, April 10, 1899

Kennedy and Roosevelt used *"vigor"* and *"vigorous"* to describe the goal we should all focus our bodies upon. They knew, as many today have forgotten, that a healthy body supports a strong and resilient mind. They also understood the consequences of a nation whose citizens became weak and unhealthy. As people seek physical comfort and ease, they inevitably avoid mental or emotional discomfort. If their goal is comfort, they avoid things that cause physical discomfort, such as exercise or healthy eating. In time, they avoid things that cause mental or emotional discomfort, such as confronting untruths or standing up for their values. It becomes easier or more convenient to let things go, whether it's their bodies or their culture. As people shirk responsibility for *themselves*, they also take less responsibility for their role in society. In time, that society unravels from within.

A great civilization is not conquered from without until it has destroyed itself from within.
   – Ariel Durant

I wrote this book for those who understand their responsibility to build and maintain a vigorous body. I hope that describes you. But I also recognize your other responsibilities outside the kitchen or gym. I want you to look, feel, and perform at your best while paying as little attention to your fitness program as possible.

Too often, I see fitness professionals whose entire lives revolve around health and fitness attempt to have clients adopt similar lifestyles. They expect clients to batch cook on Sundays, make time to eat five meals each day, go for walks in the morning, afternoon, and evening, work out, spend time in a plunge pool or sauna, fit in some yoga or meditation, and sleep for eight hours. For a young, single personal trainer who has no other responsibilities, it's possible to do it all. For a married with children middle-aged man or woman with a career, a home, and other responsibilities, doing it all is unrealistic.

I want you to do the minimum necessary to become fit and healthy. After that, if you still have time, energy, and money to invest in fitness, you can always add more. But I want you to understand how little you can do to get incredible results. To achieve exceptional health. To not become a "soft American."

Your Responsibility

In this book, I'll provide you with the knowledge and tools, but ultimately, it's up to you to put them into action. You must assume complete responsibility for your health. If you don't, you risk allowing others to assume responsibility for your illness instead.

In Kennedy's article, he further stated:

> *All of us must consider our own responsibilities for the physical **vigor** of our children and of the young men and women of our community. We do not want our children to become a generation of spectators. Rather, we want each of them to be a participant in the **vigorous** life.*

In his concluding remarks, he wrote:

> But no matter how **vigorous** the leadership of government, we can fully restore the physical soundness of our nation only if every American is willing to assume responsibility for his own fitness and the fitness of his children. We do not live in a regimented society where men are forced to live their lives in the interest of the state. We are, all of us, as free to direct the activities of our bodies as we are to pursue the objects of our thought. But if we are to retain this freedom, for ourselves and for generations to come, then we must also be willing to work for the physical toughness on which the courage and intelligence and skill of man so largely depend.

Kennedy understood that the government could not and should not control Americans. He knew that maintaining our freedom requires us to put in the necessary work to preserve our health and fitness. He foresaw that if we became gluttons and sloths, we would not only become dependent on the healthcare system for survival but also lack the stamina and strength needed to resist the tyranny that could take root in the government. His words resonate with the current state of America today.

In today's society, being fit and healthy is the exception rather than the norm. This is partly why many individuals are becoming soft, overweight, and weak. They look around and assume it's normal, that they're "not that bad." But as a collective American culture, we are indeed in a dire situation. We're increasingly unhealthy and overweight, operating at only a fraction of our potential, leaving behind a vast amount of untapped capabilities every day.

We can and should, strive for better. If not for ourselves, then for the next generations who will observe and learn from our actions. We have the choice to either lead them down a path of deteriorating health or a path that leads to the vitality and vigor that the human body was designed for.

The One Thing

About ten years ago, I read a book by Gary Keller, and Jay Papasan called *The One Thing.* I've read hundreds of business and personal development books, and none has had such a dramatic and immediate shift in the way I think about my choices each day.

The book's premise is this: In the pursuit of any goal, there's usually one thing that, if and when you do it, has a domino effect on most of the other things you need to do to reach that goal. To identify that one thing, Keller and Papasan created The Focusing Question:

> *What is the one thing I can do such that by doing it everything else will be easier or unnecessary?*

Isn't that an insightful question? Essentially, when you accomplish your "one thing," it's often a significant task that eliminates many smaller tasks. This concept proves effective in various aspects of life, including business, personal relationships, marriage, finances, and, as we'll discover, health and fitness as well.

If you were to pose that question in the context of sustaining health and fitness and enhancing longevity, the answer would be "build and maintain muscle mass." As you'll discover in the next chapter, muscle mass contributes to much more than just a sexier beach body. It impacts nearly every system in your body, including your immune, cardiovascular, and skeletal systems. Unfortunately, many people fail to grasp the significance of skeletal muscle. They live lifestyles that squander muscle, leaving them weak, frail, and sick by middle age.

I'll delve into the major benefits of muscle mass in the next chapter. However, simply being aware of its importance is not enough—you must take action to build and maintain it.

The 3 Pillars of Vigor

This is where the focusing question became even more crucial for me. I wondered, considering everything I've learned and experienced, "What is the *one thing* for building and maintaining muscle *through exercise* that, by doing it, makes everything else easier or unnecessary? And for building and maintaining muscle *through diet*? And for building and maintaining muscle *through lifestyle*?" The answers came quickly and were immediately obvious:

1. Exercise: Strength training
2. Nutrition: Protein
3. Lifestyle: Sleep

Their synergistic effect on muscle mass was clear. But then, I wondered about their synergy in dealing with common health problems or supporting health in other ways. As I delved deeper into the research, comparing their effects on the body, it became clear that those three pillars would be something worth writing a book about. You'll soon see why, if you make these three habits non-negotiable parts of your life, you won't have to invest much additional time, effort, or money into the countless other exercise programs, diets, or products available. These three pillars alone will guide you to an exceptional level of health.

That's not to say that other natural products like supplements or essential oils don't have a place in a well-rounded fitness program. I use and recommend them every day. However, they don't replace the 3 Pillars of Vigor. They may enhance your results, but they're not a low-effort, easy alternative to the pillars.

2

Muscle Mass: Health, Fitness, and Longevity.

Over the past several decades, fitness companies, magazines, and "experts" have downplayed the importance of muscle mass. By focusing primarily on its role in feats of strength and sex appeal, they've overlooked its significant impact on long-term health and longevity. Many people are unaware that in our later years, maintaining muscle mass plays a far more crucial role in health and longevity than body fat does.

Moreover, weight loss marketing and programs often overshadow the role of building healthy, functioning muscle in achieving and maintaining a lean physique. Uninformed consumers follow weight loss plans that severely reduce lean body mass and damage their metabolism. Most of the time, they end the diet and then quickly regain more body fat than they initially lost.

To fully appreciate the 3 Pillars of Vigor, you must first understand muscle mass's critical role in overall health. As you'll see, the synergy of the 3 Pillars in building muscle mass makes them indispensable to your well-being.

First, I need to explain what muscle mass really means. Then, we can explore what it does. If you prefer to skip the science, feel free to jump to the section discussing the health benefits of muscle mass.

Types of Muscle Tissue

The human body contains three types of muscle tissue: skeletal, smooth, and cardiac. Each has a unique structure and function.

1. Skeletal muscle: These muscles are attached to bones and are critical in voluntary movements. They comprise long, multinucleated fibers bundled together and surrounded by connective tissue.[6] Skeletal muscles allow us to perform various activities, from walking and lifting objects to more complex movements like dancing and playing sports.
2. Smooth muscle: Unlike skeletal muscles, smooth muscles are involuntary and found in the walls of organs and structures such as blood vessels, the digestive tract, and the uterus. They have a spindle-shaped structure and control the contraction and relaxation of these organs and structures.[7]
3. Cardiac muscle: Exclusively found in the heart, cardiac muscles pump blood throughout the body. They are involuntary and have a unique branching structure that enables the heart to contract efficiently and rhythmically.[8]

Muscle Fiber Types

This book focuses on skeletal muscle, not smooth or cardiac muscle. Skeletal muscles comprise two main types of muscle fibers: Type I (slow-twitch) fibers and Type II (fast-twitch) fibers.

1. Type I (slow-twitch): Slow-twitch fibers rely on aerobic metabolism, which means they need a steady supply of oxygen and rely on fatty acids for much of their energy. They are fatigue-resistant, making them ideal for endurance activities like long-distance running or cycling. They have a high concentration of mitochondria and myoglobin, which provide the necessary energy and oxygen for sustained muscle contractions.[9] Mitochondria are tiny organelles inside muscle cells that create energy. They're often dubbed "the powerhouses of the cells." Type I fibers can hypertrophy (grow) slightly if someone has never exercised but have less capacity to grow than Type II fibers.

2. Type II (fast-twitch): Fast-twitch fibers generate more force and are better suited for short, intense activities like sprinting or weightlifting. These fibers primarily rely on anaerobic metabolism, meaning they use a quick energy source called ATP, as well as glucose. They are more prone to fatigue than slow-twitch fibers. These fibers also have the most potential for growth.

The distribution of muscle fiber types varies among individuals and can be influenced by genetics, training, and age.[10]

Muscle Contraction

The currently accepted theory of muscle contraction is called the sliding filament theory. This theory describes the interaction between two protein filaments within muscle fibers: actin and myosin.

During muscle contraction, the myosin heads, or cross-bridges, attach to the actin filaments and pull them toward the center of the sarcomere (the functional unit of muscle fibers). This pulling action causes the sarcomere to shorten, resulting in muscle contraction. The myosin heads then detach from the actin and return to their original position, ready to repeat the process.

Energy for the contraction process comes from adenosine triphosphate (ATP), a high-energy molecule that fuels cellular processes. The myosin heads contain ATPase, an enzyme that breaks down ATP into adenosine diphosphate (ADP) and inorganic phosphate (Pi), releasing energy for the power stroke of the cross-bridge cycle.[11]

Muscle Growth and Hypertrophy

Muscle hypertrophy is the process by which skeletal muscle fibers increase in size and cross-sectional area due to resistance training or other forms of intense physical effort. Several theories attempt to explain how hypertrophy occurs. Some of the critical triggers include mechanical tension, metabolic stress, and muscle damage.

1. Mechanical Tension: Mechanical tension is created when muscles contract against an external load or resistance.

It is considered one of the primary drivers of muscle hypertrophy. Increased time under tension can lead to greater muscle protein synthesis, resulting in muscle growth.[12]

2. Metabolic Stress: Metabolic stress refers to the accumulation of metabolic byproducts, such as lactate and hydrogen ions, during high-intensity resistance training. This stress is thought to contribute to muscle hypertrophy by increasing cellular swelling and promoting anabolic (muscle or tissue-building) hormone release.[13]

3. Muscle Damage: Muscle damage occurs when muscle fibers are subjected to stress and strain during resistance exercise, causing microscopic tears in the muscle tissue. The repair and remodeling process that follows muscle damage can contribute to muscle hypertrophy.[14] However, the exact role of muscle damage in hypertrophy is still debated, with some evidence suggesting that it may not be necessary for muscle growth.[15]

4. Cellular swelling and hypoxia: Cellular swelling refers to increased muscle cell volume due to fluid accumulation during exercise. This swelling, also known as the "pump," has been suggested to contribute to muscle hypertrophy by promoting anabolic signaling pathways and satellite cell activation.[16] Hypoxia, or reduced oxygen availability in the muscle tissue, can occur during intense exercise and contribute to muscle hypertrophy. Hypoxia has been shown to stimulate the release of growth factors, such as vascular endothelial growth factor (VEGF) and hypoxia-inducible factor 1-alpha (HIF-1α), which are involved in muscle growth and regeneration.[17]

To promote continuous muscle growth, it's essential to progressively increase the demands on your muscles, a concept known as progressive overload. This can be achieved by gradually increasing your training load, volume, or intensity.[18]

The Role of Muscle Mass in Physical and Mental Health

People had admired muscular physiques throughout history, long before they understood how the body worked. Perhaps, we intuitively knew that those who were more stout, brawny, muscular, or athletic were also, on average, much healthier than the weak, soft, or frail-looking.

You'll often hear people today speak of their weak, achy, unfit physiques as products of aging. It makes for a convenient excuse. The average person's physical performance peaks in their 20s to 30s. After that, they begin losing muscle, strength, and physical performance.[19] After age 50, muscle mass and strength decline more rapidly, with strength decreasing as much as 15% per decade. We accept these numbers and ideas as reality. Yet, stats about aging come from studying what happens in the average person, and the average person becomes less active, eats a lousy diet, and neglects other essential health habits as they age. In all likelihood, people would ward off the effects of aging for years, even decades, by doing what's necessary to build and then maintain muscle mass. Here's why it's so essential.

Amino Acid Emergency Account

Have you ever had a family member experience a significant illness like heart disease, cancer, or severe COVID or flu? Chances are, their disease or condition caused rapid muscle loss. What about an injury where a limb was immobilized, or they were forced into bed rest for a while? What happened? They lost muscle. It's likely they also gained fat. Has something like that happened to you? If not, it will. It's part of living.

At 46 years old, I've experienced and come back from:

- Acute Lymphocytic Leukemia (Cancer)
- Appendicitis and an appendectomy
- Left Achilles' tendon rupture and surgical reattachment
- Left biceps tendon rupture and surgical reattachment (6 years later)
- Fractured C6 & C7 vertebrae with a severe spinal cord injury, which led to emergency anterior cervical discectomy and fusion

Illness and injuries are inevitable. You can live in fear, hiding in your home, wearing masks wherever you go, and avoiding any activity that might cause you to slip, fall, or crash. You might limit the chance of something happening, but you'd also miss out on much of what life has to offer. Alternatively, you can build up a reserve so you're ready to handle illness and injury when they happen to you.

To quickly and effectively recover, your body needs amino acids, the building blocks of protein. While you can and should eat a high-protein diet, which provides dietary sources of amino acids, you also break down muscle tissue during recovery. The more muscle you have when you get sick or hurt, the more you can afford to lose without compromising your long-term health. In this way, your muscle tissue acts like an emergency savings account.

Additionally, you'll eventually reach an age where sarcopenia, or age-related muscle loss, becomes a reality. At that time, you'll be able to slow the process with good lifestyle and nutrition choices but still lose muscle at an accelerated rate. The more you have when that process begins, the longer you'll be able to continue doing the things you love before becoming too weak to do them. In this way, muscle mass acts like a retirement or quality-of-life savings account.[20]

Blood Sugar Management and Diabetes Prevention

Insulin resistance is a significant risk factor for type 2 diabetes and is characterized by decreased responsiveness of target tissues to insulin, leading to impaired glucose uptake and utilization. According to the CDC, one in ten Americans has type 2 diabetes. One in three has pre-diabetes. By 2050, one-third of the U.S. population will have type II diabetes. One third!

Skeletal muscle is the primary site for insulin-mediated glucose uptake and is crucial in regulating glucose homeostasis. Several studies have demonstrated that higher levels of muscle mass are associated with a reduced risk of insulin resistance and type 2 diabetes.[21]

One study conducted in a large cohort of men found that higher levels of muscle mass were associated with a lower risk of type 2 diabetes, even after adjusting for potential confounding factors such as age, body mass index (BMI), and physical activity levels.[22] Another study in postmenopausal women reported similar findings, with higher levels of muscle mass associated with a lower risk of insulin resistance and type 2 diabetes.[23]

Mechanistically, increased muscle mass has been shown to enhance glucose uptake and utilization in skeletal muscle, thus improving insulin sensitivity. In addition, muscle mass is a significant determinant of resting metabolic rate. Higher muscle mass is associated with increased energy expenditure, which can help prevent obesity and reduce the risk of type 2 diabetes.[24]

Joint Protection

How many middle-aged and older adults do you know who talk about aches and pains in their joints? I would imagine you know many. Building and maintaining muscle won't wholly eliminate joint degeneration but can help slow the debilitating effects. Stronger, bigger muscles provide more support around each of your joints and help maintain proper alignment throughout your body, reducing joint stress.

If I had a dollar for every person who told me they couldn't squat because they had a bad back or knees...it would be a lot of money. Anyway, the reality is, for most people, if they'd go through the small amount of discomfort necessary to start building muscle, they'd find out that their bad knees and bad back wouldn't be bad anymore.

Though you can find some relief by using joint-supporting supplements, they play a minor role compared to strengthening your muscular and skeletal systems surrounding those joints.

Here's one more case for building joint-supporting muscle: Falls are the second-leading cause of death from unintentional injuries, next to auto accidents.[25] When you fall, the strength of the muscles surrounding your joints can determine whether your fall leads to a serious injury or not. If you're strong enough, your muscles brace your joints and minimize the pain and injury. If you're weak and you fall, you're more likely to break.

Inflammation Reduction

Systemic inflammation causes numerous health problems, including cardiovascular disease, cognitive decline, and joint degeneration. Low muscle mass is correlated with higher inflammation levels. In this way, muscle mass acts like an organ, regulating inflammation and acting as part of your immune system.[26]

Maintaining Metabolic Rate

Muscle costs your body a lot of energy. That's why it gets rid of muscle you don't use. But as long as you use it consistently, your body will maintain the muscle despite the energy required. In doing so, it'll look for energy elsewhere, such as your body fat.

By investing a small amount of time each week, following a well-designed strength and conditioning program, eating a high-protein diet, and getting enough sleep, you tell your body it needs more muscle. As long as you keep giving it the signal, it'll respond by increasing the size of your muscle cells, thereby improving your metabolic rate. If you burn more energy at rest, keeping your body fat levels in check will be much easier.

Look Healthier

Muscle makes you *look* healthier. I'm often surprised by the number of healthcare practitioners, and even some fitness professionals, who don't look strong and healthy. Many are overweight or obese and are supposed to influence others toward better health. That's not to say that you should judge a fitness professional based on his or her looks alone. There are plenty of personal trainers and health coaches who post daily, almost-naked selfies as a way to attract clients. Many of them might look the part on the outside but have little to offer regarding real-world experience or sound knowledge. But, I digress.

When you're stronger and more muscular, you carry yourself differently. You maintain a better posture. And as you carry yourself differently, you start to feel differently. If you look sloppy, you'll feel sloppy, and others will be more likely to see you as sloppy. If you look strong, you'll feel strong, and others will be more likely to see you as a strong person.

Protect Your Heart

Research suggests that people with greater muscle mass have a lower risk of cardiovascular disease and related complications. A study published in the *Journal of the American College of Cardiology* found that higher muscle mass was associated with a lower risk of cardiovascular disease in men and women. The study involved over 6,000 individuals and concluded that muscle mass might protect against cardiovascular disease, independent of other factors such as age, sex, and body mass index.[27] Other large-scale studies have come to similar conclusions.[28,29]

A 10-year study followed men and women without any sign of cardiovascular disease at the beginning.[30] Not surprisingly, men in general were more likely to develop cardiovascular disease. What stood out, though, was that **those with the highest levels of muscle mass were the least likely to develop cardiovascular disease. They were 81% less likely to have a heart attack or stroke.**

Enhance Cognitive Function and Brain Health

Maintaining muscle mass may also positively impact cognitive function and overall brain health. A study of older adults found that greater muscle mass was associated with better cognitive performance, as measured by tasks assessing attention, memory, and executive function.[31] One possible explanation for this association is insulin-like growth factor 1 (IGF-1), a hormone produced in response to resistance training and muscle growth. IGF-1 has neuroprotective effects and is involved in the growth, differentiation, and survival of neurons in the brain.[32]

Bigger Is Better

Bigger is better. At least, it is when it comes to muscle mass. In the following three parts of the book, I'll review The 3 Pillars of Vigor. Ultimately, the goal is to leverage these three pillars to build muscle for as long as possible, and once you're no longer able to build more, to maintain it as long as possible.

As powerful as the three pillars are for building muscle, you'll see how synergistic they are for helping you improve overall health and fitness and, potentially, improve longevity.

II

Pillar 1: Strength Training

If you think lifting is dangerous, try being weak.
Being weak is dangerous.
– Bret Contreras

3

Healthy Training

Some people will skip this part of the book or perhaps not even purchase it due to its inclusion. They might prefer being told that walking is a sufficient form of exercise, or that following a yoga video on YouTube will suffice. Alternatively, they might convince themselves that playing pickleball is adequate. While I enjoy pickleball as well, it simply cannot compare to the benefits of resistance training.

Regrettably, I've even heard fellow fitness professionals advise people to "Do whatever type of exercise you enjoy," as if all exercise is equal. You'd dare not tell people to think like that about food or much else in life. Doing just what feels good rarely has good long-term outcomes. I understand why fitness professionals give such bad advice; they don't want to offend anyone and desire to be liked by all. However, my priority is helping people achieve results, even if it means conveying information that some may not want to hear.

You might be surprised I'm stressing resistance training without saying a word about cardio. Many people have been led to believe that cardio is the ultimate form of exercise for health, but that's mainly due to marketing tactics rather than the actual health advantages it provides.

Let me be clear: cardio isn't necessarily bad. However, it *can* cause muscle loss, contribute to overuse injuries, compromise muscle growth, and sometimes even lower testosterone levels and contribute to cardiovascular issues. On the other hand, resistance training is undeniably more beneficial and essential.

If someone wants to incorporate cardio into their routine, and they have the time for it *in addition to* their strength training without hindering their overall fitness results, then they should go for it. But in most cases, strength training should be the priority.

Note: The one exception to my strength training first recommendation is for women with PCOS. Research and experience have shown that they benefit more from frequent cardio and less frequent strength training. Generally, those with PCOS tend to see better results with two days of resistance training per week and four to five days of cardio, especially when paired with a ketogenic diet. But that's a specific case and a topic for another book or blog post.

Now, let's dive into the impressive benefits you'll gain from committing to regular strength training sessions.

Blood Sugar and Insulin

When healthy people consume carbohydrates, their blood sugar (glucose) rises, prompting insulin secretion. Insulin signals the liver and muscle tissue to store glucose within their cells. The liver fills up first and has limited storage capacity. Muscle cells soak up the remaining glucose, provided they have enough space. If the muscle cells are full or don't respond to insulin's signal to store the glucose, glucose accumulates in the bloodstream, eventually converting into fat. Meanwhile, insulin levels remain elevated until blood sugar returns to normal.

Blood glucose spirals out of control when:

1. You consistently consume more carbohydrates than can be stored as glycogen or used through physical activity.
2. Your muscles have room to store carbohydrates, but the cells stop responding to insulin signals. This is called insulin resistance.

Contracting muscles primarily burn adenosine triphosphate (ATP) and glycogen. Exercise, therefore, utilizes some stored glycogen, creating space for more. Intense strength training sessions can deplete glycogen stores by 24-40%.[33] Moreover, consistent resistance training can enhance insulin sensitivity.

More Americans suffer from insulin resistance (prediabetes) or full-blown Type II diabetes than those who don't. The solution to this health issue is clear to those who understand basic physiology, yet many remain uninformed. The majority of the US population has insulin resistance or Type II diabetes, an epidemic that extends to much of the Western world. By 2050, if trends remain the same, one-third of the US population will have Type II diabetes.[34] I should also point out that Alzheimer's disease, which is becoming ever more common as well, is often dubbed Type III diabetes because of its connection to insulin resistance and blood sugar.

Belly fat contributes to insulin resistance and diabetes. Consistent resistance training programs can decrease belly fat, subsequently reducing insulin resistance.[35]

The truth is, strength training is the most crucial activity for diabetics and anyone serious about avoiding insulin resistance or diabetes.

Fat Loss

Most people likely associate exercise for reducing body fat with cardio—hours on a treadmill, elliptical, or stationary bike. Some might even think signing up for a marathon and starting to run is the answer. However, cardio is generally unnecessary for most people to achieve a healthy body composition, with the exception being women with polycystic ovary syndrome (PCOS). Excessive cardio can increase inflammation levels, and chronic inflammation contributes to numerous degenerative diseases.

After completing a study, David Nieman, a professor at Appalachian State Univerisity and pioneer in the research area of exercise and nutrition immunology, stated, "The immune system reflects the stress the body goes through during long-distance running... After every long run, the immune system is heavily occupied with repairing muscle damage. Stress hormones increase as glycogen levels decrease, contributing to transient inflammation and immune dysfunction."[36]

Excessive cardio can also cause muscle tissue breakdown, reduced testosterone and thyroid hormones, elevated cortisol, and overuse injuries. One study even discovered a concerning link between marathon running and heart disease. While it's possible to list more reasons why excessive cardio might be a poor choice for most people, the point should be clear.

In contrast, a meta-analysis of 58 studies demonstrated that resistance training significantly impacts body fat reduction.[37] Long-term, it helps lower body fat by raising metabolic rate as you increase muscle mass, and by controlling blood sugar as you increase the capacity for storing glycogen. But in the short term, a good strength training session stimulates fat metabolism immediately, as well.

Catecholamines and Lipolysis

Catecholamines, such as norepinephrine and epinephrine, stimulate receptors in fat cells, which enhances insulin sensitivity, lowers blood sugar and insulin levels, and increases fat metabolism.[38]

You may recall the popularity of ephedrine as a fat loss supplement in the early 2000s. It was effective because ephedrine stimulated adrenergic receptors in fat cells, the same receptors needed for epinephrine and norepinephrine to have their effects. However, it also allegedly increased the risk of cardiovascular events, leading the FDA to ban it.

Overloaded muscle tissue, similar to what is experienced during a hypertrophy-style strength training session, produces a comparable effect. When muscles are overloaded, they release microRNA 1 (miR-1) containing extracellular vesicles (EVs). Epididymal white adipose tissue (eWAT) then absorbs these EVs, which in turn increases B-adrenergic (AdrB3) expression and promotes lipolysis (fat breakdown). The elevated catecholamine levels also increase overall energy expenditure, allowing fatty acids to be utilized for energy and ultimately reducing fat mass.

Increased Glycogen Storage and Reduced Blood Sugar

When you consume carbohydrates, they are typically used in one of four ways:

1. Burned for immediate energy needs
2. Stored in liver and muscle cells as glycogen
3. Left to circulate in the bloodstream, causing damage as seen in people with type II diabetes
4. Converted to triglycerides and stored as fat

For most people, it's unlikely to eat a meal's worth of carbohydrates and burn them off immediately. As a result, the latter three scenarios are more common. This is where resistance training plays a crucial role. As mentioned in the previous section, having more muscle mass increases your carbohydrate storage capacity. Consequently, when you consume carbs, you have somewhere to store them, preventing elevated blood sugar levels and minimizing the conversion of carbs into fat.

Improved Strength and Stamina

Weak bodies often become more sedentary, and in turn, sedentary bodies lead to weaker bodies. To break this downward cycle, it's crucial to engage in activities that are physically demanding, like weight training. Building muscle and stamina through resistance training makes it easier to carry out everyday activities.

The more strength and stamina you have, the more time you'll spend on your feet rather than sitting. Conversely, being sedentary reduces energy expenditure and contributes to insulin resistance. This leads to elevated insulin levels and makes it harder to burn fat effectively.

Increased Metabolic Rate

Strength training results in micro-trauma within your muscle cells. This microscopic muscle damage triggers your body to build more muscle, a process that demands energy.[39] Consequently, your metabolic rate stays elevated during the recovery period. Research indicates that your metabolic rate remains significantly higher for up to 24 hours after a training session.[40] This increased energy expenditure and a greater reliance on fat for fuel mean you burn more fat even while resting between workouts.

Hormones

Strength training enhances the production of human growth hormone (HGH), a hormone responsible for growth, cell reproduction, and cell regeneration.[41] This hormone is instrumental in maintaining and improving muscle mass, bone density, and overall health. By engaging in regular strength training, we can effectively slow down the aging process and maintain the vigor of youth.[42]

Testosterone, another hormone positively affected by strength training, plays a crucial role in the development of muscle mass, bone density, and a plethora of other vital functions.[43] Both men and women can experience a boost in testosterone levels through regular weightlifting, which ultimately increases strength, energy, and overall well-being.

Moreover, strength training has been shown to reduce cortisol levels - the infamous stress hormone.[44] By providing our bodies with a healthy outlet to relieve stress, we actively contribute to our emotional well-being.

Cardiovascular Health

Strength training depletes oxygen in the blood. Without oxygen, your contracting muscles produce lactate, which causes your muscles to burn. Your heart beats harder and faster to remove lactate and deliver more oxygen to your working muscles.

Continued strength training sessions lead to improvements in stroke volume and a reduction in resting heart rate, which means your heart becomes more efficient. Research also demonstrates that resistance training positively impacts the health of your blood vessels. Although some healthcare practitioners caution hypertensive patients against resistance training, this advice contradicts research findings. A 2017 meta-analysis revealed that when hypertensive or pre-hypertensive patients participated in a strength training program, both diastolic and systolic blood pressure decreased over time.[45] Blood pressure may increase slightly during exercise but drops quickly after completing a set, ultimately having a positive effect on blood pressure overall.

One study summarized the cardiovascular benefits of strength training in this way: "High levels of muscular strength appear to protect hypertensive men against all-cause mortality, and this is in addition to the benefit provided by cardiorespiratory fitness."[46]

Coordination, Mobility, and Pain Relief

In a study conducted on nursing home residents with a mean age of 89 years, a 14-week resistance training program led to a 60% increase in average strength and a gain of more than three pounds in lean mass.[47] Imagine the impact this program had on their coordination and mobility! And think about how much it could improve an elderly person's quality of life!

Strength training enhances the quality of your movement by boosting strength around your joints. It also improves your mobility, which is the ability to move through a greater range of motion while your muscles are contracted. For instance, hamstring mobility enables you to bend over and pick something up from the floor without compromising your back's position.

With better-coordinated movement, you move more powerfully and can safely react to unexpected terrain. Moreover, moving with improved coordination and enhanced mobility makes you less likely to experience chronic joint pain. One of the most exciting outcomes for my clients over the years has been their significant reduction, if not elimination, of pain.

Bone Density

According to the Bone Health and Osteoporosis Foundation:[48]

- A woman's risk of fracture is equal to her combined risk of developing breast, uterine, and ovarian cancer.
- Men are more likely to suffer a bone fracture due to osteoporosis than to be diagnosed with prostate cancer.
- A quarter of hip fracture patients aged 50 and older die within a year of the fracture.

- Six months after a hip fracture, only 15% of patients can walk across a room without assistance.

Dense bones support your weight when you jump, trip, or slip on the ice. The lower your bone density, the more likely you are to suffer a fracture.

Resistance training serves as a stimulus for bone density, just as it does for muscle mass. Provided you consume enough protein, magnesium, vitamins D and K, and calcium to build bone, your body should experience consistent improvement in bone mineral density once it receives the signal from your strength training sessions.

Myokines

This effect of muscle deserves special attention, though it's a little more technical than the previous benefits we've reviewed. You see, muscle acts like a secretory organ, not just a tissue for moving your body. The effects of the compounds secreted from movement and exercise have a profound effect on your health. It's little wonder that the more we sit, the sicker we get.

When your muscles move, they secrete chemical messengers called cytokines, which directly affect how your brain functions and influence other bodily systems. You might be familiar with the term "cytokine" from the media attention on COVID-19 in recent years. "Cytokine storms" occurred in some patients, leading to severe illness and even death.[49] These cytokines controlled inflammation, which spiraled out of control and resulted in multi-organ failure and death in some cases. Some people also experienced cytokine storms after receiving a COVID-19 vaccine.[50]

To clarify, the cytokines I'm discussing in relation to the mental and physical health benefits of exercise are not the same as those that cause harm. Many of the body's cytokines are anti-inflammatory, and even pro-inflammatory cytokines are essential for metabolic function, although they can become problematic when things go awry.[51]

Muscle cell contraction produces a specific category of cytokines called myokines.[52] Myokines may affect the muscle cells themselves (an autocrine effect), nearby cells (a paracrine effect), or cells far away from them (an endocrine effect).[53] Interestingly, you secrete different myokines when you train with higher loads and fewer reps than when you train with lower loads and higher reps,[54] further emphasizing the importance of a professionally designed program that incorporates varying rep ranges.

The following are the most important myokines released during and after strength training:

Brain-Derived Neurotrophic Factor (BDNF)

As the name suggests, BDNF stimulates the growth and development of neurons. It also enhances memory and learning, ultimately affecting cognitive function.[55] This fact alone should lead people to demand that gym classes are a staple in public schools and nursing homes. In addition to its positive effect on the brain, BDNF:

- aids in the recovery of damaged muscle tissue[56]
- enhances fat metabolism in muscle cells[57]
- improves glucose utilization, helping to normalize blood sugar levels[58]

Myostatin

Myostatin reduces muscle cell growth, meaning low myostatin levels lead to greater muscle growth.[59] In humans, it's extremely rare for someone to maintain low myostatin levels, but strength training does help to lower myostatin levels temporarily, allowing for increased muscle growth.[60]

The Belgian Blue bull is the best example of what happens when myostatin levels are minimized. These bulls are born with a genetic trait that shuts down myostatin production. As a result, they're far more muscular than a typical bull.[61] Google the images of these incredible creatures. If animals could compete in bodybuilding, Belgian Blue bulls would be the winners.

People with muscle wasting diseases, myopathy, or sarcopenia often have high levels of myostatin, but they also tend not to perform much resistance training.[62] It's possible that consistent resistance training would help lower myostatin, allowing them to preserve muscle mass.[63] As of yet, there is no pharmaceutical solution for lowering myostatin, which makes resistance training all that much more important.[64]

Decorin and Follistatin

Decorin and Follistatin are myostatin antagonists, meaning that they compete with the effects of myostatin, which helps lead to muscle cell growth.[65,66] Decorin also enhances myoblast (undeveloped cells that can become muscle cells) proliferation and inhibits angiogenesis and tumorigenesis (tumor formation).[67] Follistatin stimulates satellite cell proliferation, may enhance the healing of injured muscles, and reduces muscle scar tissue formation.[68,69]

Interleukin-6 (IL-6)

Interleukin-6 (IL-6) is often seen as a pro-inflammatory cytokine. For example, the havoc created by a cytokine storm is, at least in part, due to high levels of IL-6.[70] Interestingly, when muscle cells secrete IL-6, it lowers inflammation levels.[71] Following an intense strength training session, IL-6 levels can rise by up to 100 times.[72] IL-6 also:

- inhibits TNF alpha and IL-1 beta[73]
- improves insulin sensitivity[74]
- stimulates satellite cell proliferation, which helps cause muscle cell growth[75]
- stimulates protein synthesis[76]
- increases levels of anti-inflammatory biomarkers and reduces levels of inflammatory biomarkers[77]

Irisin

Irisin is a hormone that promotes the conversion of white adipose tissue to brown adipose tissue, which is more metabolically active and thermogenic.[78] This leads to increased energy expenditure and improved fat metabolism. In addition to its fat-burning effects, Irisin also:

- Enhances bone density[79]
- Reduces insulin resistance and improves glucose utilization[80]
- Crosses the blood-brain barrier, stimulating the secretion

of BDNF in the brain, which enhances cognitive function[81]
- Stimulates cancer cell death (apoptosis)[82]
- Aids in mitochondrial biogenesis, contributing to the growth and maintenance of healthy mitochondria[83]

Meteorin-Like (Metrnl)

Meteorin-like, also known as Metrnl, is a recently-discovered myokine that contributes to the conversion of white adipose tissue to brown adipose tissue, leading to improved insulin sensitivity.[84] Although research on Metrnl is still in its early stages, it holds promise for further understanding its role in metabolism and overall health. Current studies suggest that Metrnl is involved in immune response and inflammation regulation.[85]

Meterorin-like also causes the conversion of white adipose tissue to brown adipose tissue, which enhances insulin sensitivity. This is one of the most recently-discovered myokines, so there's much more to learn about it.

Myokines and Program Design

We can effectively stimulate myokine secretion by manipulating variables such as rep ranges, loads, and other program design elements. Training with lower rep ranges (1–5) and heavier loads suppresses myostatin and increases decorin, stimulating muscle growth or hypertrophy. In contrast, higher rep ranges (10–15) and lighter loads promote the secretion of BDNF and irisin, enhancing our cognitive function, neuroplasticity, and metabolic health.[86,87] By varying rep ranges and loads, we can strategically influence the release of these myokines to optimize our body's response to resistance training.

Another key variable in program design is the rest intervals between sets. Shorter rest periods (30-60 seconds) have been associated with a more significant increase in interleukin-6, a myokine with both pro- and anti-inflammatory properties, which is essential for muscle repair and regeneration.[88] Longer rest periods (2-5 minutes), on the other hand, can lead to a more pronounced release of meteorin-like, a myokine involved in enhancing insulin sensitivity and reducing inflammation.[89]

Mental Health

Strength training has been shown to improve mood and reduce symptoms of depression. A meta-analysis of 33 clinical trials found that resistance training effectively reduced depressive symptoms in adults, regardless of age, sex, or the improvement in muscle strength.[90]

The exact mechanisms behind this mood enhancement remain unclear, but it is hypothesized that strength training may increase the production of endorphins, serotonin, and other neurotransmitters that contribute to positive mood states.[91]

Building and maintaining muscle mass through strength training can also help improve stress resilience and reduce anxiety. A systematic review of 16 studies found that resistance training significantly reduced anxiety symptoms in both healthy individuals and those with a physical or mental health diagnosis.[92]

Resistance training may help modulate the stress response by promoting the release of brain-derived neurotrophic factor (BDNF), a protein that supports the growth and survival of neurons and plays a role in stress resilience.[93]

Summary

The benefits of resistance training are truly far-reaching, touching upon nearly every aspect of human physiology and overall health. It is unfortunate that strength training is not more widely emphasized in school physical education programs or in fitness offerings for senior living communities and nursing homes. As you've seen, strength training has a profound impact on both physical and mental health, going beyond just building muscle mass to improving cognitive function, insulin sensitivity, and bone density, among many other benefits.

With a new appreciation for the importance of resistance training in your life, it's time to explore what strength training entails and how to differentiate effective programs from mere entertainment.

4

What is Strength Training?

What is Strength Training?

If you ask 100 people their idea of strength training, you'll get 100 very different answers. The primary purpose of a resistance training workout is to create stress within your muscle cells. That stress leads to an adaptation. Of course, for our purposes here, we want them to grow larger and stronger, so I'll mainly focus on resistance training with that goal in mind. However, you should also experience a significant increase in muscular endurance and stamina, especially if you're not strength training already.

Progressive Overload

Understanding and applying the principle of progressive overload is essential for an effective resistance training program. The story of Milo of Croton, an Italian wrestler from around 500 B.C., illustrates this concept. Milo began by carrying a newborn calf on his shoulders and continued to carry it as it grew into a bull. As the calf became heavier, Milo's strength increased.

This tale demonstrates the simplicity of building muscle and strength: you must continually overcome greater physical force than you have in the past. There are various ways to progressively overload your muscles, but arguably the most effective and easiest to understand is by increasing the weight you use for different exercises. For example, if you're doing back squats with a barbell on your back, you might start with only the 45-pound bar for two sets of 12 repetitions each. The following week, you could add five-pound plates to each side of the bar and complete two sets of 12 reps with 55 pounds. This progression exemplifies progressive overload.[94]

In your first few months of strength training, you should experience significant improvements due to neurological adaptations. As you become more comfortable with various exercises, you'll develop greater coordination and use more of your existing muscle mass. Eventually, you'll reach your strength threshold with your current muscle mass. By continuing to push yourself to use heavier loads, you'll stimulate muscle growth.[95]

In general, you'll use progressive overload in your strength training program to:

1. Lift heavier weights than you have in the past for the same number of reps you've handled previously. Example: Last week, you did ten bodyweight squats. This week, you do ten bodyweight squats while holding 10-pound dumbbells in each hand.[96]
2. Use the same weight while lifting it for more reps than you did in the past. Example: Last week, you did ten

bodyweight squats. This week, you do 15 bodyweight squats.[97]

3. Perform more total sets for an exercise, which increases the total volume. Example: Last week, you did one set of 10 bodyweight squats. You did two sets this week; next week, you'll do three.[98]

The essential point to understand is this: resistance training sessions never get easier. You become more comfortable with the effort you must put into them, but they don't get "easier." You may experience some weeks that feel easier than previous weeks, particularly when transitioning to a new training cycle of exercises. However, to maintain progress, you must continue to work harder over time.[99]

Just as your work becomes more challenging as you get better at it, making you even better, your workouts become more difficult as you get fitter, further improving your fitness. You have to "do the work," which I often remind my clients of. Embrace the challenge, stay consistent, and remember that progress takes effort and dedication.

SAID Principle

A second, equally important principle you should understand is the SAID Principle, an acronym for Specific Adaptation to Imposed Demands.[100] The idea is that your body adapts to specific stressors, which makes you more capable of handling similar stressors in the future. The principle applies to learning, skill development, how your immune system develops immunity, or how your skin tans in response to the sun.

Of course, we're most concerned here with developing strength and muscle mass. For example, you shouldn't expect to build muscle while training for a marathon. Marathon training breaks muscles down. It causes your body to favor smaller, slow-twitch muscles over stronger, bigger, fast-twitch muscles.[101] Low-resistance, high-repetition exercise, like many group fitness classes, also compromises muscle size and strength, favoring muscular endurance.

You can use a number of different variables to trigger increases in strength and muscle mass, including sets, reps, rest periods, training volume, time under tension, training frequency, and a bunch of other advanced training techniques. For most people, it's best to keep things simple, changing as few variables as possible to get good results. When designing programs for most of my clients, I vary only the following variables:

1. Reps: The number of repetitions you complete for an exercise before taking a rest.
2. Sets: The number of times you perform an assigned number of reps for an exercise.
3. Load: The weight or resistance that's applied against you during an exercise.
4. Exercise: To hit all the major muscle groups effectively, you need to incorporate various forms of presses, pulls, squats, deadlifts, and some rotational movements. A minor change to an exercise, such as doing reverse lunges instead of walking lunges, can be enough of a new stimulus to produce significant results.

Unfortunately, many programs add in other variables and

complexity, such as supersets, triple sets, and compound sets, or they have clients complete a ridiculous number of reps for a given exercise, which compromises the muscle and strength benefits and also increases the risk of injury.[102] Such techniques can be powerful tools when used appropriately but can be counterproductive for the average adult.

Basics of a Good Strength Training Program

The following are general guidelines I use in designing programs for my clients. They're not set in stone, and I do veer from these guidelines in a given 12-week training block as I consider how that 12-week block fits within the year's entire program. Also, if you're a beginner, I might have you do less than what's listed below.

40-60 Minutes per Session

I didn't write this book for athletes or bodybuilders taking steroids. I wrote it for average adults who have a life outside the gym. You don't need to spend more than an hour on resistance training, but you do need more than the 15 minutes some ad on social media suggests. Most training sessions should take 40-60 minutes, including your prep work at the beginning.

About Ten Sets per Body Part per Week

While there's some individuality in this, research shows that completing ten sets per week per body part works well for stimulating muscle growth.[103] For "body parts" I'm referring to the major movers; legs, chest, back, shoulders, arms, and calves. Not to get sidetracked in minutia, but I noted calves in the list, a muscle group most people ignore. Yet, training your calves not only strengthens them but also improves mobility, which then affects your ability to squat or even walk normally.

You could complete all ten sets in a single workout once per week or divide them over 2-3 workouts during the week. The more sets you try to fit into a given workout, the fewer body parts you can train during that workout. If you tried to hit all body parts in a workout with ten sets each, you'd be in the gym for hours, which goes against the first guideline above.

6-20 Reps per Set

The more reps you try to complete, the less weight you'll be able to use. During some training blocks, I'll have clients use fewer reps and focus on developing strength, and in others, I'll have them use higher reps for their sets. Most of the time, though, I use a mix of both high and low rep ranges or keep most of the sets in the middle, like 8-15 reps. If I designed a program for specific athletes, I might choose other rep ranges, but this works best for most people looking for optimal health, fitness, and longevity.

Divide Body Parts Over Two to Three Workouts

I've never been much of a fan of "full-body" workouts, where you complete at least one exercise for each body part and then do two to three workouts per week. I've found that, as you get in better shape and try to train near your limits of strength, fatiguing your entire body gets brutal on your nervous system.

Training in a way that hits only part of your body in a workout improves body composition and stimulates muscle growth without beating down your nervous system.

You can divide your body up in numerous ways, but the three most common I use in my programming are:

1. Upper / Lower: Chest, Back, Shoulders on Monday and Thursday, and Legs and Arms on Tuesday and Friday.
2. Push / Pull: Thighs, Chest, Shoulders, and Calves on Monday and Thursday, and Back, Biceps, and Abdominals on Tuesday and Friday.
3. Legs / Back & Chest / Shoulders & Arms: In this training split, you'd do legs on Monday, Back, and Chest on Tuesday, and Shoulders and Arms on Thursday. Friday, you'd start the cycle again.

There are many ways to mix up these training splits as well. Of course, the goal is to get results, not to change the program for your entertainment constantly.

Do 3-6 Workouts Before Changing Routine

Without question, one of the most misguided pieces of advice any trainer has ever said is, "you need to keep changing things up and keep your body guessing." This notion is still being passed around from one fitness enthusiast to another, but in reality, it's far from accurate.

Remember, you need progressive overload to build strength and muscle. You must work harder than you did the previous week. The most effective way to ensure you do this is to complete the same training session with more reps or weight than you did before. If you change your workouts every week, you can't be sure you'll push yourself harder. At that point, you must rely on your perceived exertion, which is always subjective and unreliable.

5

Getting Started

What to Expect

As you begin training, your strength increases in three stages, with the final stage leading to muscle growth.

Improved Coordination

It feels awkward the first time you try to do a new exercise. You won't have good coordination. Each time you do it again, you get better and stronger. Once you have mastered the coordination for the movement, you can handle much more weight. Each week, you may add 10, 20, or even 30 more pounds to the weight you can handle for the exercise.

This is common in all movements, especially with novice lifters. Once you've developed coordination, your nervous system starts using more of the muscle you already have.[104]

Nervous System Engagement

You have enough strength to lift a car off a child trapped underneath it. However, your nervous system prevents you from using that kind of strength because you'd do significant damage to your muscle tissue, ligaments, and tendons. The bragging rights of lifting a car won't be worth it if you're confined to a hospital bed for months afterward. That said, you can lift more weight safely than your nervous system allows in the early stages of strength training.

By repeating the same movements over time, your nervous system realizes it can handle more weight without injury, so you gain significant strength without building more muscle.[105]

Muscle Growth

Unfortunately, most people don't make it to the third stage. It takes time and consistency. If you keep at it, you'll reach a point where your strength gains slow. But if you keep training hard, you'll force your body to make you stronger still. The only way to do that in this stage is to build more muscle.

As I often tell my clients, if you want to get results, you need to commit for the long term and remain monogamous to your fitness program. If you play the field with various programs, you'll likely end up disappointed by the results, leading to the all too common excuse, "Nothing ever works for me." Don't cheat on your program with other programs.

Assuming you don't give up, you should start seeing actual muscle growth within 3–6 months. As your muscle grows, you begin experiencing the health benefits of muscle, as covered in part one. But along the way, you also experience the health benefits of your actual strength training sessions.

Getting Started with Strength Training

It can feel daunting to start strength training. When you get to the gym, which exercise do you start with? How do you perform the exercise? How do you include enough exercises to hit each muscle group often enough to get results but not too often so you're constantly sore?

A lot of fitness books include a recommended workout program inside the book. I thought about doing that, too. The problem is, no matter how detailed it is, the workouts always appear more complicated in writing than they are when they show up in an app.

So, instead of having you read about a workout program, I'd like to give you the experience. Assuming you've never trained with me before, you can pick one of the following programs and get it for free for a month. If you like it, you can keep going with my membership program, which costs a tiny fraction of what one-on-one personal training in a club would cost.

Choose the one that program that best suits your needs and preferences. If you enjoy it, you can continue training with me. If not, or if you'd like to use the free month to understand how a professional program feels, you can cancel any time during your first month, and it won't cost you anything. I believe this is the best way for you to experience the recommendations I've made throughout this chapter and start reaping the numerous health benefits of strength training. To register for your program of choice, go to tomnikkola.com/3-pillars/bonus.

1. Intro to Resistance Training: Build strength and improve

body composition while gaining an understanding of how your muscles should feel during training. Using primarily machines, this beginner program provides extra stability and guides you through the proper range of motion, boosting your confidence in performing the exercises correctly.

2. Genesis (Intro to Free Weights): This beginner program helps you gain confidence and comfort in performing essential free weight exercises for developing strength, mobility, and physical stamina. Experience increased lean muscle mass, strength, and a youthful look and feel. Most clients who complete Genesis transition to either Vigorous or Resilient.

3. Resilient: Designed with middle-aged women in mind, this intermediate/advanced program focuses on building conditioning and stamina that make you leaner and fitter and help you handle the stress and pressure of everyday life. Resilient includes more conditioning or cardio than Vigorous.

4. Vigorous: Tailored for middle-aged men, this intermediate/advanced program prioritizes strength training to help you build visible muscle and gain the strength and stamina needed to tackle even the most challenging tasks. Vigorous includes occasional conditioning work.

If you have the opportunity to work with a one-on-one trainer, go for it. It can be a significant investment, but if you work with an experienced trainer and follow his or her program, even when you're not with them for a workout, I'm certain it'll be worth it. But, if you don't have a trainer available, or it doesn't fit in the budget, I'd love to have you try one of my training programs. Remember, go to tomnikkola.com/3-pillars/bonus to access your program of choice.

III

Pillar 2: Protein

When life gives you lemons, ask for something higher
in protein
– Unknown

6

High-Protein

I grabbed the skin fold calipers to measure the body fat on the back of her arm. As I gently separated the muscle from the fat to get an accurate measurement, I was surprised at how much fat I held. The caliper reading confirmed my surprise.

The woman, dressed in street clothes, appeared healthy and slim in her t-shirt and workout pants. We'd already discussed the sixty pounds she had lost but not the diet she'd followed to achieve it. "Have you been doing Weight Watchers?" I asked. She turned her head to look at me, curious. "How did you know?" she inquired.

Her example was all too common and still is today. Low-calorie, low-protein weight loss plans, especially those that don't incorporate resistance training, cause considerable muscle loss. This is especially true for women, who have less muscle mass than men, on average, to begin with. Weight Watchers was one of the most common of such programs at the time.

Despite anti-meat-eating propaganda, the truth is that many Americans don't consume enough protein for optimal health.[106] Research and my experience indicate that a high-protein diet would benefit most people. That's why a high-protein diet is Pillar 2.

What is a High-Protein Diet?

As I explained in Chapter 2, amino acids are the building blocks of protein, and your muscle tissue is made of protein. You need to eat protein to supply your body with the amino acids necessary for muscle growth and all the other roles amino acids play.

The Recommended Daily Intake for protein is 0.8 grams per kilogram of body weight.[107] According to the RDI, that is an "adequate amount for most people to avoid deficiency."[108] Adequate to avoid deficiency? Is that what we should aim for? It seems that's the case for most people. The RDI is well below optimal. And while most Americans eat right around the RDI, almost half of older adults don't even meet this level.[109]

A high-protein diet is primarily defined by the increased consumption of protein-rich foods, which support various bodily functions, including muscle growth and repair, immune response, and hormone production. While the exact percentage of daily caloric intake from protein may vary, it typically ranges from 20% to 35%, or even higher in some cases. This contrasts with the standard American diet, where protein intake typically accounts for around 15% of total calories.[110]

The high-protein diet also contrasts other popular diets, such as low-carb, ketogenic, and low-fat. I felt it was worth reviewing how the different diets are identified.

1. Low-carb diet: A low-carb diet emphasizes a reduced carbohydrate intake, often accounting for less than 30%

of total daily caloric intake.[111] The focus is on consuming more protein and fat while limiting foods high in sugars and starches. While a high-protein diet can also be low-carb, the primary distinction is that a low-carb diet specifically targets a reduction in carbohydrate intake.

2. Ketogenic diet: The ketogenic diet is a very low-carb, high-fat diet where the primary goal is to induce a metabolic state called ketosis. In this state, the body uses ketones, derived from fat, as an energy source instead of glucose, which comes from carbohydrates.[112] The macronutrient distribution for a ketogenic diet typically consists of 70-80% fat, 20-25% protein, and 5-10% carbohydrates. While both high-protein and ketogenic diets may share similarities in reduced carbohydrate consumption, a ketogenic diet focuses on increasing fat intake to promote ketosis, rather than primarily increasing protein intake.

3. Low-fat diet: A low-fat diet restricts dietary fat consumption, often limiting it to 20-30% of total daily caloric intake.[113] The diet encourages the intake of carbohydrates and protein to compensate for reduced fat consumption. A high-protein, low-fat diet may emphasize lean protein sources, such as poultry, fish, and plant-based options. Still, the key distinction is that a low-fat diet specifically focuses on minimizing fat intake, whereas a high-protein diet emphasizes increased protein-rich foods.

High-protein diets can be identified and quantified using different approaches. The most common methods include defining protein intake based on a percentage of total daily calories, a specific amount per kilogram of body weight, or a specific amount per pound of body weight. Let's take a closer look at each of these approaches:

1. Percentage of total daily calories: In this approach, a high-protein diet is defined by the proportion of protein intake relative to the total caloric intake. As mentioned earlier, a high-protein diet typically consists of 20% to 35% or more of total daily calories from protein sources. This is higher than the standard American diet, where protein intake usually accounts for around 15% of total calories. To calculate protein intake based on this method, you would first determine your total daily caloric needs, then multiply that number by your desired protein percentage.

2. Grams of protein per kilogram of body weight: Another standard method to define a high-protein diet is by setting specific protein intake goals based on an individual's body weight. The recommended daily allowance (RDA) for protein is 0.8 grams per kilogram of body weight.[114] However, for a high-protein diet, the protein intake is typically higher, ranging from 1.2 to 2.2 grams per kilogram of body weight, depending on factors such as activity level, age, and health status.[115] To calculate protein intake using this method, you would multiply your body weight (in kilograms) by your desired protein intake (in grams per kilogram).

3. Grams of protein per pound of body weight: This approach is similar to the previous one, but it uses pounds instead of kilograms for measuring body weight. The RDA for protein using this method is around 0.36 grams per pound of body weight. For a high-protein diet, the recommended range is between 0.55 and 1.0 grams of protein per pound of body weight, depending on factors such as activity level, age,

and health status. To calculate protein intake using this method, you would multiply your body weight (in pounds) by your desired protein intake (in grams per pound).

The first option has limitations because your protein intake would depend on your total calories consumed. If your calories are low, your protein will inevitably be low, too. On the other hand, if you're an athlete who needs several thousand calories per day, your protein goal would be much higher than necessary. That's why I prefer the second or third option, which bases your protein target on your body weight. Protein targets stay the same and you can modify your carbs or fat based on your calorie needs (if you're tracking calories).

As I live in the United States, I'll refer to pounds and grams here, such as method three describes. Assuming you don't have preexisting kidney disease, there is no real risk in consuming too much protein, but it is possible to eat too little. Based on both anecdotal and scientific evidence, the ideal target for protein intake appears to be about 1 gram of protein per pound of goal body weight for men, and between 0.8-1.0 gram of protein per pound of goal body weight for women.

With that in mind, as we continue reviewing Pillar 2, please understand that we're discussing a high-protein diet of at least 0.8 grams per pound of goal body weight for women and at least 1.0 grams for men. As you'll see, those Americans eating at or below the RDI are missing out on the numerous benefits of a higher-protein diet. While consuming more meat may not be politically correct, it is physiologically correct.

7

High-Protein Health Benefits

High-protein diets don't just help you look better. They also impact your overall health. The following are some of the most significant ways high-protein diets enhance your well-being.

Better Mental Health

Research shows that a high-protein diet can reduce depression and anxiety symptoms. A randomized controlled trial investigated the effects of a high-protein diet on depression symptoms in overweight and obese adults. Participants were assigned to either a high-protein or a standard-protein diet for 12 weeks. The participants in the high-protein group had a more significant reduction in depression symptoms than those in the standard-protein group.[116]

Another study investigated the effects of a high-protein diet on anxiety symptoms in women. The women were assigned to either a high-protein or a low-protein diet for ten weeks. The results showed that participants in the high-protein group had a more significant reduction in anxiety symptoms than those in the low-protein group.[117]

Research has also suggested that a high-protein diet can improve mood and cognitive function. A study investigated the effects of a high-protein diet on mood and cognitive function in healthy adults. Participants were assigned to either a high-protein or a normal-protein diet for seven days. The results showed that participants in the high-protein group had improved mood and cognitive function compared to those in the normal-protein group.[118] And lastly, a meta-analysis of studies on those who avoid eating meat showed that meat abstainers (i.e., vegans, vegetarians) had significantly higher rates of depression, anxiety, and self-harm behaviors.[119]

Overall, research suggests that a high-protein diet may be beneficial for reducing depression and anxiety symptoms and improving mood and cognitive function. However, more research is needed to fully understand the relationship between a high-protein diet and mental health.

Fat and Weight Loss

You've undoubtedly been led to believe that weight loss is all about creating a calorie deficit. Fitness magazines, the media's "health experts," and the government's dietary guidelines repeat this misleading concept repeatedly, even though research doesn't support it. The makeup of your diet—the macronutrients—plays a more significant role in how your diet affects your body composition than the calories it contains.

When calories are kept the same between two groups, the group that eats more protein experiences better improvements in body composition.[120] They lose more body fat and maintain or even gain muscle tissue.[121]

In another study design, participants follow an *ad libitum* diet. They must eat a set protein level but get no other dietary recommendations.[122] In this study, higher protein intake also favors better body composition.[123]

When working with clients on their nutrition, I first recommend increasing protein intake. I don't care what other carbs and fat they eat as long as they eat more protein. They almost always consume fewer carbs and less fat without thinking about it and get leaner without feeling like they're on restrictive diets. High-protein diets:

- **Increase satiety:**[124] Protein stimulates the release of cholecystokinin, PYY, and GLP-1, which reduce feelings of hunger and increase satiety, prolonging the length of time before hunger returns.[125] The hormones alter signals in your brain about food needs.[126] This can be crucial as it relates to breakfast. High-protein breakfasts reduce cravings for junk food later in the day, including for children.[127]

- **Fill you up faster during a meal:** By eating more protein, you'll unconsciously eat less fat and carbohydrate. This is even more effective if you eat all your protein at the beginning of your meal.

- **Stimulate diet-induced thermogenesis:** Though it's a small metabolic difference, you burn about five times as many calories digesting and assimilating protein as you do fat or carbohydrate. For every 100 calories of protein you eat, your body burns about 25 calories to digest and absorb it. In comparison, your body only burns about 8-10% of carbohydrates and 3-5% of fat.[128]

Not only is a high-protein diet more effective for weight loss, it's also more effective for keeping the weight off once you've lost it. Many people rebound after reaching their goal weight, but a high-protein diet can help you maintain a leaner body once you've achieved it.[129] Even after a year, those on a higher protein diet and without specific calorie goals, are more likely to maintain their weight loss.

Unsurprisingly, a high-protein diet combined with a good resistance training program is superior for improving body composition.[130]

Muscle Mass

A higher protein diet combined with a well-designed strength training program builds muscle while you're young enough to build it and enables you to maintain it as you reach later adulthood.

Your level of muscle mass can be a better predictor of longevity than your body fat level.

Dietary protein or branched-chain amino acids stimulate protein synthesis and slow protein breakdown. Research shows a high-protein diet can cause a slight increase in muscle mass if you don't exercise at all. Of course, the effects will be more significant when combined with weight training.

Bone Health

Based on almost 42,000 women, the lower one's protein intake, the higher the risk of hip fractures. High-protein diets stimulate calcium absorption, bone turnover, and insulin-like growth factor 1 (IGF-1) production.[131] IGF-1 stimulates osteoblast activity. Osteoblasts secrete the matrix for bone formation. Integrative health doctors also use IGF-1 as a reference for growth hormone, one of the essential hormones for supporting muscle mass and fat metabolism.

Protein also positively affects parathyroid hormone, which affects bone health.[132] While dietary protein increases calcium absorption, it can also increase calcium secretion.[133] Eating vegetables and taking calcium, magnesium, and vitamins D and K would counteract that loss. Still, the bottom line is that research shows higher-protein diets have a positive effect on bone health, not a negative one.[134]

Blood Sugar

Slight elevations in blood sugar are normal. Significant short-term increases or even small but chronic increases in blood sugar may lead to insulin resistance and diabetes. What drives up blood sugar more than anything else? Dietary carbohydrates.

Not surprisingly, high-protein diets improve body composition and lower blood sugar.[135] That shouldn't be a surprise, but increasing protein consumption also lowers blood sugar even when someone eats a higher-carb diet or even foods high in *sugar.*

I have to tell you about one particular study that, even with as much as I knew about protein already, still blew my mind. Researchers compared the impact of consuming only protein-rich shakes multiple times each day to an equal-calorie, normal-protein, whole-food diet. The total calories were the same between the two diet groups, but the high-protein diet group consumed 211 grams of protein per day, while the control group consumed 83 grams (about the same as the average American consumes each day). But, along with the protein variations, the researchers threw in a few other major differences.

1. The high-protein group consumed only 4 grams of fiber per day. Meanwhile, the control group consumed 92 grams of fiber per day.
2. The shake used for the high protein group was made with soy protein. I wouldn't recommend consuming soy protein, especially that much. I'd also expect whole food to have a more significant effect than protein powder of any sort.
3. The high-protein group consumed 179 grams of *sugar* per day. ONE HUNDRED SEVENTY-NINE GRAMS! Not only is that an absurd amount of sugar, but it would likely send the participants' blood sugar through the roof and limit any fat-burning benefits from the higher protein intake, right? Let's see.

The study participants spent 32 hours in a whole-body calorimetry unit (WBCU), the most accurate and expensive way to track metabolic rate measures. You have to live inside this small room all by yourself so that it can measure temperature changes based on the heat your body produces. Using this calorie-measuring technique long-term isn't practical, but it's the most accurate method available.

Compared to those following a normal diet, the high-protein group:

- Increased their daily calorie expenditure and post-meal metabolic rate, and experienced better sleep
- Increased fat metabolism and **decreased carbohydrate**

usage even though they consumed 179 grams of sugar!
- Decreased blood triglycerides

Despite consuming almost no fiber, a ridiculous amount of sugar, and using soy protein instead of a higher-quality protein source, the higher-protein group experienced much better effects from their diet than the other group during that short study.

Stress

When you're under stress, your body uses more protein to combat cortisol's effects and support your immune system.

Many people who start exercising, or begin a weight loss program, get sick shortly after getting started. It's often because they add the stress of the diet or exercise without eating sufficient protein to support their immune system and other metabolic needs.

Whenever I can get through to someone who is "always sick," I encourage them to increase their protein intake. It's incredible to see how quickly they get over their illness.

Healthy, resistance-trained men followed a diet for two weeks that was designed to match 60% of their usual calorie intake.[136] One group ate a high-protein, low-fat diet, and the other ate a moderate-protein, moderate-fat diet. The higher-protein group experienced less fatigue, more satisfaction with the diet, less stress, and less mood disturbance than the moderate-protein group.

Immune Function

A high-protein diet can have numerous benefits for the immune system. It has been suggested that protein is necessary for maintaining optimal immune function as it is required to produce immune cells, enzymes, and antibodies. Additionally, protein can improve immune response by increasing the production of cytokines, which are signaling molecules that play a key role in regulating the immune system. Remember, we talked about the role of cytokines in the chapter about strength training health benefits.

A study published in the *Journal of Nutrition* found that a high-protein diet, when combined with regular exercise, increased the number of immune cells in the body, including lymphocytes, which play a critical role in fighting off infections.[137] Another study published in the *American Journal of Clinical Nutrition* found that a high-protein diet enhanced the immune response in healthy adults, resulting in greater resistance to infection.[138]

Moreover, a high-protein diet can also improve wound healing and reduce inflammation, which is essential to maintaining a healthy immune system. A study published in the *Journal of Wound Care* found that increasing protein intake improved wound healing in elderly patients with pressure ulcers.[139] Similarly, another study showed that a high-protein diet reduced inflammation in obese individuals, potentially reducing their risk of chronic diseases.[140] Insufficient protein intake makes people more susceptible to infection as well.[141]

Cardiovascular Health

One study found that a high-protein diet can help lower blood pressure in adults with pre-hypertension and hypertension.[142] The study participants who consumed a diet high in protein for 12 weeks showed a significant decrease in systolic and diastolic blood pressure compared to those who followed a standard diet. The researchers suggest that this effect may be due to the blood pressure-lowering effects of some amino acids found in protein, such as arginine and lysine. Another study showed that blood pressure also dropped by adding protein supplements to the diets of overweight adults.[143]

Another study found that a high-protein diet can improve blood lipid profiles, an essential factor in reducing the risk of cardiovascular disease.[144] The study participants who followed a high protein diet for six months showed a significant decrease in triglyceride levels and an increase in high-density lipoprotein (HDL) cholesterol levels compared to those who followed a standard diet. The researchers suggest that this effect may be due to the ability of high-protein diets to increase satiety, reduce calorie intake, and improve insulin sensitivity.

Do You See What I See?

Are you starting to see how incredible the effects of a high-protein diet are on human health? And you can make this dietary change without any restrictions at all!

Most of the time, when people think about changing their diet, they start to think about all the stuff they need to stop eating. I don't want you to do that. The moment I tell you to *stop* eating something is the moment you want to eat more of it.

I'm suggesting there's a benefit to eating *more*, at least more protein. And by doing so, you'll likely eat less of other stuff without telling yourself you need to stop eating. You'll stop eating because you'll get full faster and stay full longer.

Before moving on to how you get started with a high-protein diet, I want to address some frequently asked questions. You'll find them helpful, especially if you talk to other people about increasing your dietary protein.

8

Common Questions & Concerns

Inevitably, when I teach, write, or post about protein, people respond with pushback based on myths dispelled long ago. The following questions and answers cover the most common ones.

What if I overeat protein?

You might be afraid of overeating protein if you believe in the myth that your body weight depends solely on managing calories. The fact is, you *will not* gain body fat by overeating protein. The only thing that's likely to happen is that you'll feel full longer after meals than you otherwise would.

Dr. Jose Antonio and his team divided 30 men and women into two groups to verify this.[145] Ten served as a control group, and 20 were put in a high-protein group, consuming **two grams of protein per pound of body weight** per day. That's twice as much as the "1 gram per pound goal body weight" target I suggested as optimal. The extra protein they ate was in addition to their maintenance calorie level, which meant they increased their daily calories by about 800. According to the calorie balance

76

equation, this should have caused them to gain 1.6 pounds of fat per week. By the end of the eight-week study, the high-protein group gained...nothing. The extra protein and calories did not affect their body fat levels.

In another study, the same research group overfed men and women with 1.5 grams per pound bodyweight of protein and put them on a heavy resistance training program.[146] In this study, although they were in a calorie surplus due to the higher protein intake, they dropped body fat and increased lean body mass.

The bottom line is this: Eating extra protein will not be detrimental, so long as you don't have pre-existing kidney disease. In fact, it may accelerate your fat loss and muscle-gaining goals.

What kind of protein is best for me?

Whey protein is, hands down, the best protein source for a supplement, based on research to date. Hundreds of research papers back it up. I recommend including a high-quality whey protein shake or two in your daily nutrition practice whenever possible, especially if you're having difficulty eating enough protein through food alone. If you tolerate lactose, whey concentrate is fine. If you don't, look for whey isolate. Personally, I rely on food most of the time and an occasional whey-based protein bar.

For food, animal protein is superior in its effect on our health, but some people refrain from animal products, which I respect. Vegetarians and vegans must be more intentional about consuming optimal levels, including supplementing with protein powders.

Is there a minimum or maximum I can eat at a meal?

This is only a loose guideline. For women, I'd suggest shooting for at least 30 grams per meal at a minimum. For guys, I'd recommend at least 40 grams per meal. From there, it just depends on how many meals you eat. To trigger protein synthesis (muscle growth), you need a minimum amount of essential amino acids, specifically leucine. Consuming at least 30-40 grams of high-quality protein should meet that threshold to stimulate protein synthesis.

Since you're shooting for a daily intake, you can loosely divide your protein needs by the number of meals you eat. I usually eat two or three meals, so I split my daily intake over those three meals, with dinner generally being the biggest meal.

As for a maximum, once you've consumed 30-40 grams of high-quality protein, you no longer stimulate higher levels of protein synthesis (muscle growth). However, muscle catabolism (breakdown) continues to slow with higher and higher intakes. The extra protein may be used for other functions, as well. The point is, there's not a "maximum" amount for a meal, though at a certain point, you just won't be able to eat anymore.

What should I do if I'm vegetarian or vegan?

Find a way to increase your protein intake without using starchy carbohydrate sources. You'll probably have to drink at least a few plant-based protein shakes daily. It'll be a lot easier if you're vegetarian and willing to eat dairy, eggs, or even fish.

If I'm an older adult, do I need less protein?

You need more protein. As you age, your body doesn't respond to protein as well, an aging process called "anabolic resistance." You must eat more protein for the same muscle-stimulating (anabolic) response you would have gotten when you were younger by eating less. I would also suggest using digestive enzymes and possibly hydrochloric acid, as enzyme and HCl production also decrease with age. These enzymes and acids help with the breakdown and assimilation of protein.

Do I have to time my protein with exercise?

Timing isn't that important unless you are a high-performing athlete who has to be super-fine-tuned with his or her food and supplements. Just eat it when you can. You might hear "experts" say that you must eat within an hour of exercise, but again, if you're not a professional athlete, it doesn't matter. They're just regurgitating out-of-date advice.

What if I have an allergy or sensitivity?

Then don't eat that protein source. Find something different.

What if I don't like to eat protein?

You have a choice. Eat something you don't like as much, so you can enjoy how you look and feel as your body changes, or eat what you want and dislike how you look and feel.

What if it's not grass-fed, pasture-raised, or wild-caught?

Do your best with what's available and what you can afford. I'm often surprised by the number of people who refuse to eat animal protein that isn't grass-fed beef, pasture-raised pork, or wild-caught fish and then eat organic junk food. Eat the best sources, but don't let a less-than-ideal source or protein keep you from eating it. When we travel, I'm happy to buy jerky and protein shakes at the gas station or eat chicken or turkey from the deli counter if that's what works.

9

How to Get Started

If you currently consume the average amount of protein for Americans, approximately 98 grams per day for men and 68 grams for women, you don't need to reach your "1 gram per pound of ideal body weight" target immediately. Gradually increase your daily intake each week for several weeks, and you'll be close to your optimal amount within a month or so. This gradual approach is often how I assist clients in working towards a consistent high-protein diet.

Start With Your First

If you eat breakfast, begin there. Women, aim for at least 30 grams of protein, and men, aim for at least 40 grams of protein at breakfast. You can eat more but don't eat less. Keep it simple, or you won't stick with it. An easy option is an egg scramble with some frozen vegetables and deli meat. A protein shake is another alternative. Leftovers from the night before serve as a third option.

Eat Protein First

Always prioritize eating your protein first, whether it's a snack or meal. This practice helps you trigger your satiety signals more quickly, fills your stomach with denser food, and ensures you consume all of your protein before getting sidetracked by carbs and fat.

Research indicates that even when people eat the same food, consuming protein first leads to a slower rise in blood sugar and less insulin release than if they ate their carbs first. In one study, subjects consumed ciabatta bread and orange juice first, followed by grilled chicken breast and a lettuce and tomato salad.[147] On a different day, they reversed the order, eating the chicken and salad first. When consuming their protein and vegetables first, their blood glucose levels were 28.6%, 36.7%, and 16.8% lower at 30, 60, and 120 minutes after eating! So, make it a point to eat your protein first.

Eat Enough, Then Worry About Quality

If it's accessible and affordable, choose higher-quality animal protein sources such as grass-fed meat, pasture-raised poultry, pork, eggs, and wild-caught fish. However, don't avoid animal protein sources that don't meet such high standards if that's all that's available to you.

I recall being on a cruise with hundreds of other health-conscious travelers. I overheard some of them in the cafeteria lamenting that the meats, poultry, and fish didn't meet their high standards and that they'd resort to eating salads and starches for the week. It was challenging not to chuckle at their predicament.

As mentioned earlier in this chapter, the most crucial aspect is consuming enough protein. If you can achieve this while eating only the finest protein sources, that's fantastic. However, if you can't, it's better to eat something that may not be the absolute best in terms of quality to ensure you get enough total protein for the day.

Keep It Simple

When discussing current nutrition habits with people, most realize that they tend to eat pretty much the same foods from one week to the next. However, when they decide to start a new "diet," they suddenly feel the need for recipes and food ideas as if they're entirely lost. The perceived need for recipes can be an unconscious attempt to overcomplicate matters, providing an excuse for not following through. You don't need a new cookbook. Just start cooking—meat and vegetables seasoned with a little dry spice. It's that simple.

Many people stumble over the belief that every day has to offer something different. It doesn't—especially for breakfast or lunch. For several years while working at Life Time's corporate office, my lunch consisted of the same cycle of meals, unless I dined out. You can try this approach too.

Purchase 1 pound each of ground chicken, turkey, beef, bison, and lamb. Then, pick up a few different frozen vegetable blends, such as California blend, Mediterranean blend, and stir-fry blend. Each evening, brown 1 pound of the meat, mix in your choice of vegetables, and add your choice of dry seasoning. Transfer the mixture to a glass container, cover it, and you have 1-2 meals for the next day.

Keep it simple—because simplicity is key to sticking with it.

10 Example High-Protein Meals

Since I'd expect someone will ask, I've listed ten high-protein meals below. You might notice I didn't use eggs or cottage cheese in the example meals. That's not because I'm against eating them, I just didn't use them in the example meals. So, if you add some meals with eggs or cottage cheese, you'll have even more options.

Each meal has about 500 calories and 60 grams of protein, so increase or decrease your portion size based on your needs.

1. Grilled Chicken Breast Salad: Grilled chicken breast (200g) with mixed greens (100g), cherry tomatoes (50g), cucumber (50g), avocado (50g), and balsamic vinaigrette. Calories: 525, Protein: 60g.

2. Baked Salmon with Sweet Potato: Baked salmon (200g) with roasted sweet potato (150g) and steamed broccoli (100g). Calories: 555, Protein: 60g.

3. Beef Stir Fry: Sautéed beef (150g) with mixed vegetables (150g) such as bell peppers, onions, and mushrooms, served over brown rice (50g). Calories: 585, Protein: 60g.

4. Shrimp Scampi: Sautéed shrimp (200g) with garlic, butter, and lemon juice, served over zucchini noodles (150g). Calories: 555, Protein: 60g.

5. Roasted Pork Tenderloin: Roasted pork tenderloin (200g) with roasted carrots (100g), brussels sprouts (100g), and sweet potato (100g). Calories: 585, Protein: 60g.

6. Greek Yogurt Parfait: Greek yogurt (250g) with mixed berries (100g) and granola (25g). Calories: 550, Protein: 60g.

7. Turkey Chili: Ground turkey (200g) with kidney beans

(100g), diced tomatoes (50g), onion (50g), and chili seasoning, served with cornbread (50g). Calories: 580, Protein: 60g.

8. Tuna Salad Sandwich: Tuna (150g) mixed with mayo and diced celery, served on whole wheat bread (50g) with lettuce and tomato. Calories: 560, Protein: 60g.

9. Steak Fajitas: Sautéed steak (150g) with bell peppers (50g) and onions (50g), served with salsa, sour cream, and whole wheat tortillas (50g). Calories: 570, Protein: 60g.

10. Chicken Curry: Chicken breast (200g) cooked in a curry sauce with coconut milk and vegetables such as bell peppers, onion, and carrots, served over rice (50g). Calories: 595, Protein: 60g.

So far, we've covered strength training as a means of stimulating muscle growth and eating more protein as a way to provide the building blocks to build it. Now, we need to talk about the perfect environment for building muscle and supporting a vigorous body. Let's move on to Pillar 3.

IV

Pillar 3: Sleep

No aspect of our biology is left unscathed by sleep deprivation.
– Matthew Walker

10

Sleep, Muscle, and Health

"What can I do to boost my testosterone?" It's one of the most common questions I get from middle-aged guys. "Why do you think you have low testosterone?" I ask. The most common response was, "I lost my libido." My next question is, "How many hours of sleep do you get each night?" More often than not, the answer is less than seven.

These guys aren't low in testosterone. They're living in sleep debt. Some people don't get enough hours of sleep. Others, whether it's due to medications, alcohol consumption, stress, or the heat of their bedroom, don't get into deep and REM sleep when they do sleep. Either way, about half of adults live in sleep deprivation.[148]

Sleep is a critical component of the muscle growth and recovery process. During sleep, the body undergoes physiological and hormonal changes that facilitate muscle repair, growth, and overall recovery. Below, we'll explore some key aspects of the connection between sleep, muscle growth, and your physical and mental health.

Hormones

During sleep, particularly in the deep stages of non-rapid eye movement (NREM) sleep, you get a surge in the production of anabolic hormones, such as growth hormone (GH) and insulin-like growth factor 1 (IGF-1).[149] Growth hormone stimulates protein synthesis, cell regeneration, and overall tissue growth, while IGF-1 promotes muscle growth by increasing amino acid uptake and protein synthesis in muscle cells.[150]

In contrast, sleep deprivation or poor-quality sleep can lead to a decrease in anabolic hormones and an increase in catabolic (muscle or tissue-destroying) hormones, such as cortisol, which can impair muscle recovery and growth.[151]

Muscle Protein Synthesis

Adequate sleep is essential for optimal muscle protein synthesis, the process through which the body repairs and builds muscle tissue. Research has shown that sleep deprivation can negatively affect muscle protein synthesis by reducing the activation of mTOR signaling, a crucial pathway in regulating muscle growth.[152]

Furthermore, a lack of sleep can decrease the efficiency of dietary protein intake in stimulating muscle protein synthesis.[153] This means that even with an adequate protein intake, sleep debt makes your body less able to use it.

Immune Function

Sleep also plays a vital role in maintaining a healthy immune system. During sleep, the body produces cytokines, which are proteins that regulate immune and inflammatory responses.[154] Adequate sleep ensures the proper functioning of the immune system, which is essential for muscle recovery and growth.

Cardiovascular Health

Sleep plays a vital role in maintaining optimal cardiovascular health. During sleep, the body undergoes several restorative processes, including blood pressure regulation, heart rate modulation, and inflammation reduction. A growing body of evidence suggests that sleep duration and quality are closely linked to cardiovascular health outcomes, with sleep disturbances and disorders posing a considerable risk for cardiovascular diseases (CVDs).

A seminal study by Cappuccio et al. demonstrated a strong association between short sleep duration (less than 6 hours per night) and an increased risk of developing coronary heart disease and stroke. The study, which involved a meta-analysis of 15 prospective studies, revealed a 48% increased risk of developing or dying from coronary heart disease and a 15% increased risk of stroke in individuals with short sleep duration.[155]

Moreover, sleep apnea, a sleep disorder characterized by repetitive interruptions in breathing during sleep, has been linked to an increased risk of developing hypertension, arrhythmias, and heart failure. In a review by Drager et al., the authors found that sleep apnea is an independent risk factor for CVD, with a four-fold increase in the risk of myocardial infarction, stroke, and death from CVDs.[156]

Additionally, poor sleep quality has been associated with an increased risk of CVD. Difficulty falling asleep, frequent awakenings, and non-restorative sleep are all independently associated with an increased risk of acute myocardial infarction.[157]

Blood Sugar and Insulin

Studies have shown that sleep deprivation can negatively impact glucose metabolism and insulin sensitivity, increasing the risk of developing type 2 diabetes and other metabolic disorders.[158]

During sleep, our bodies undergo several restorative processes, including regulating blood sugar levels. Inadequate sleep can disrupt these processes, leading to an increase in blood glucose levels. One study found that restricting sleep to just four hours per night for six nights resulted in a 40% reduction in glucose tolerance and a 30% decrease in insulin sensitivity.[159]

Another study observed that individuals who reported sleeping less than six hours per night had a higher risk of developing impaired fasting glucose, which can be a precursor to type 2 diabetes.[160] Moreover, research showed that one week of sleep restriction (to five hours per night) led to a 20% decrease in insulin sensitivity in healthy adults.[161]

Insulin sensitivity is important because it determines how effectively our bodies can use insulin to lower blood sugar levels. Reduced insulin sensitivity, or insulin resistance, can cause glucose to build up in the bloodstream instead of being absorbed by cells for energy. Over time, this can lead to type 2 diabetes.[162]

Body Fat and Weight Management

Sleep significantly impacts weight gain, even when caloric intake is controlled. Numerous studies have shown a strong connection between sleep duration, quality, and weight gain.[163] The primary reason for this link can be attributed to the influence of sleep on hormones and metabolism, which regulate appetite and energy expenditure.[164]

One key hormone affected by sleep is leptin, produced by fat cells and responsible for telling your brain that you are full.[165] When you don't get enough sleep, your body produces less leptin, leading to an increased appetite and a decreased ability to feel satiated.[166] Conversely, sleep deprivation also leads to higher ghrelin levels, a hormone that stimulates hunger. These hormonal imbalances can contribute to weight gain even if caloric intake is kept in check.

In addition to hormonal effects, sleep plays a crucial role in regulating glucose metabolism and insulin sensitivity.[167] Inadequate sleep can lead to insulin resistance, making it more difficult for the body to process glucose and increasing the risk of developing type 2 diabetes.[168] Insulin resistance can also contribute to weight gain, as it promotes fat storage in adipose tissue.[169]

Moreover, poor sleep quality can impact energy expenditure and the body's ability to burn calories. Sleep deprivation can lead to feelings of fatigue and reduced motivation to engage in physical activities, ultimately leading to a more sedentary lifestyle.[170]

Gut Health and the Microbiome

Studies have shown a strong connection between the quality and quantity of sleep we get and the state of our gut microbiome – the diverse community of trillions of microorganisms that live in our digestive system.[171] These microbes help with digestion, nutrient absorption, immune system function, and even the production of neurotransmitters that influence our mood and cognition.[172]

One study by researchers at the University of Colorado Boulder found that just two nights of partial sleep deprivation led to significant changes in the gut microbiome, including a decrease in the abundance of beneficial bacteria.[173] This disruption in the balance of gut microbes, also known as dysbiosis, has been linked to various health issues such as obesity, inflammatory bowel diseases, and even mental health disorders like anxiety and depression.[174]

Sleep deprivation can also increase the levels of the stress hormone cortisol, which is known to affect the gut by reducing the production of mucus that protects the gut lining, thereby making it more susceptible to inflammation.[175] Inflammation in the gut can further disrupt the microbiome balance and create a vicious cycle that impacts overall health.

On the other hand, maintaining a healthy sleep pattern can promote gut health. A study published in the journal *Nature Communications* showed that individuals with a regular sleep routine had a more diverse gut microbiome than those with irregular sleep patterns.[176] The research suggests that establishing a consistent sleep schedule can positively influence the gut microbiome and improve overall health.

Mental Health

Sleep is crucial in maintaining mental health, affecting various aspects such as mood, cognitive function, and overall psychological well-being.[177] When we consistently get sufficient quality sleep, our brain can perform essential tasks like memory consolidation and emotional regulation.[178] In contrast, inadequate sleep can lead to several negative consequences on our mental health.

Firstly, sleep deprivation increases the risk of developing mood disorders such as depression and anxiety.[179] A study published in the journal *Sleep* revealed that individuals who reported sleep problems were more likely to develop depression later in life.[180] Additionally, people with anxiety disorders often have difficulties falling asleep or experience frequent awakenings throughout the night.[181] This bidirectional relationship between sleep and mood disorders suggests that addressing sleep issues could help improve mental health outcomes for many individuals.

Moreover, chronic sleep loss can impair cognitive functions such as attention, memory, and decision-making.[182] Research has shown that sleep deprivation can lead to decreased alertness, slower reaction times, and diminished problem-solving abilities.[183] Sleep is essential for memory consolidation, as it helps to solidify and organize the information we have learned throughout the day.[184] Consequently, sleep deprivation significantly compromises your ability to learn and retain new information.

In addition to mood disorders and cognitive impairment, poor sleep exacerbates stress symptoms and contributes to burnout. Studies have shown that individuals with poor sleep quality experience higher levels of stress and a reduced ability to cope with daily challenges.[185] By negatively impacting our ability to manage stress, sleep deprivation can further compromise our mental health and overall quality of life.

Furthermore, sleep disturbances are often observed in individuals with post-traumatic stress disorder (PTSD) and other trauma-related disorders.[186] Research has indicated that disrupted sleep can worsen symptoms of PTSD, as well as impede the recovery process.[187] Addressing sleep issues in individuals with trauma-related disorders is crucial for promoting healing and improving mental health outcomes.

Sleep also plays a vital role in the regulation of emotions. A lack of sleep can lead to increased emotional reactivity and a reduced ability to regulate negative emotions.[188] This emotional dysregulation can exacerbate existing mental health issues and create difficulties in interpersonal relationships, further contributing to psychological distress.

Pain Sensitivity

Sleep plays a crucial role in maintaining good overall health, and its relationship with pain sensitivity is a topic of growing interest among researchers. Studies have found that adequate sleep can help modulate pain perception, while sleep deprivation may increase pain sensitivity.[189]

A study conducted by Krause et al. investigated the link between sleep and pain by inducing sleep deprivation in healthy participants.[190] They discovered that those who were sleep-deprived displayed increased pain sensitivity, as evidenced by lower pain thresholds and higher pain intensity ratings. This suggests that even short-term sleep loss can significantly impact our perception of pain.

The role of neurotransmitters and hormones in the body can partly explain the connection between sleep and pain sensitivity. During sleep, the body releases anti-inflammatory cytokines and growth hormones, which can help repair damaged tissues and reduce pain.[191] Additionally, sleep is essential for proper functioning of the endogenous pain-inhibitory system, which involves the release of neurotransmitters like serotonin and dopamine. These chemicals help modulate our perception of pain, and disrupted sleep can affect their levels.[192]

Furthermore, sleep and pain sensitivity are influenced by a bidirectional relationship. Chronic pain can cause sleep distur-bances, while inadequate sleep can worsen pain or contribute to new pain. This creates a vicious cycle that can be difficult to break, making it essential for individuals suffering from chronic pain to prioritize good sleep hygiene.

Libido or Sexual Desire

A lack of sleep or poor sleep quality can lead to decreased sexual desire, while a consistent, healthy sleep pattern can help improve it. Sleep affects libido in several ways, including its impact on hormone regulation, stress levels, and mood.

One of the main ways sleep affects libido is through hormone regulation. Sleep is essential for maintaining a balance of hormones, including testosterone and estrogen. Testosterone, in particular, is a critical hormone for both men's and women's sexual desire and function.[193] Studies have shown that testos-terone levels tend to increase during sleep, especially during rapid eye movement (REM) sleep, and decrease with sleep deprivation.[194] Consequently, consistently getting a good night's sleep can help maintain healthy hormone levels and support sexual health.

Another factor to consider is the impact of sleep on stress levels. Chronic stress can lead to a decrease in sexual desire.[195] Insufficient sleep, in turn, can exacerbate stress and anxiety, further contributing to a lowered libido.[196] By improving sleep quality and quantity, you may experience reduced stress levels, positively influencing libido.

Lastly, sleep has a significant impact on mood. Sleep disturbances like insomnia have been linked to depression and mood disorders.[197] Depression can negatively affect libido, often resulting in a lack of interest in sex.[198] Ensuring a regular and healthy sleep schedule can help improve mood and sexual desire.

Summary

We all experience inadequate sleep now and then, but after reading this chapter, I hope your eyes are open to chronic sleep deprivation's devastating effects on your health. I've worked with many people who've had many different health issues. Some had difficulty with gut health, others had no libido, and some men hadn't had a morning erection since they were in college. Others had trouble building muscle or were always sick. Still others were forgetful or depressed. And still others had trouble losing weight, despite the fact that they trained hard and ate well. All had one related underlying cause: sleep deprivation. In the next chapter, we'll get into how you can significantly improve the quantity and quality of your sleep.

11

Getting Enough

Now, for the good news: most people live in sleep debt by choice. They choose to stay up too late, watching shows, scrolling through social media, or working well beyond the hours necessary for their job. Many have even convinced themselves that they're "night owls" because they've trained themselves to stay up late at night. Since you live in sleep debt by choice, you can also choose not to live in sleep debt. Your body and brain will thank you in the years to come.

How much sleep do you need?

The National Sleep Foundation provides the following recommendations:

- Older adults (65+): 7-8 hours
- Adults (18-64 years): 7-9 hours
- Teens (14-17 years): 8-10 hours
- School-age children (6-13 years): 9-11 hours
- Preschoolers (3-5 years): 10-13 hours

- Toddlers (1-2 years): 11-14 hours
- Infants (4-11 months): 12-15 hours
- Newborns (0-3 months): 14-17 hours

How do you measure up against these recommendations? And how about other people in your family? By understanding your sleep needs and making a conscious effort to prioritize rest, you can make a significant positive impact on your overall health and well-being.

Remember, these are ranges for the average person. I often tell my clients they need 7+ hours of sleep every night. That doesn't mean they're good to go if they get exactly seven hours. Some people would feel, look, and perform much better if they consistently got eight hours. Not to mention that when people aim for seven hours, they often get only six and a half hours by the time they fall asleep.

When you short yourself on sleep, you damage your body and contribute to cognitive decline. This is because your body and brain receive special, separate treatment during sleep, with one phase of sleep supporting tissue repair and another contributing to cognitive health, learning, and memory formation.

By prioritizing sleep and ensuring that you consistently achieve the recommended hours for your age group, you'll improve your physical health and support your mental well-being. Sleep is an investment in your overall quality of life, so make it a priority and experience the benefits of a well-rested body and mind.

Sleep Phases

Your body is a remarkable machine governed by an internal clock that orchestrates the delicate dance of hormones and neurotransmitters, guiding vital processes such as sleep, wakefulness, and physical activity. At the core of this intricate system lies the suprachiasmatic nucleus (SCN), a cluster of cells in your brain that acts as the master conductor of your body's rhythms.[199]

Yet, the environment also plays a pivotal role in influencing your circadian rhythm, the natural 24-hour cycle that regulates your sleep-wake patterns. External factors that impact your circadian rhythm are known as Zeitgebers.[200] Light is the most potent Zeitgeber, but other factors, such as diet, exercise, and supplementation, can also sway the SCN and your overall well-being.[201]

Disturbing your circadian rhythm can have serious consequences for your health. A prime example is the 25% surge in heart attack rates observed on the Monday following the shift to Daylight Saving Time.[202] This single-hour change in schedule highlights the profound impact that even minor disruptions can have on our bodies, raising questions about the necessity of Daylight Saving Time in today's world.

Under normal circumstances, your circadian rhythm guides you through three distinct sleep phases each night.

Light Sleep

During light sleep, you find yourself in a state of semi-consciousness. You maintain awareness of your surroundings, responding to unexpected stimuli such as the creaking of a door or the whisper of a loved one. While your mind can still process these events, your body remains relaxed and disinclined to move unless provoked by a perceived threat or an irresistible urge.[203]

Under the weight of significant stress, you may spend a disproportionate amount of time in this light sleep stage, depriving yourself of the restorative benefits offered by the subsequent phases.[204] Ideally, light sleep lasts for 10-30 minutes before you naturally transition to the more rejuvenating deep sleep stage.[205]

Deep Sleep

Deep sleep is critical for your body's growth, repair, and overall well-being. During this stage, the production of growth hormone reaches its peak, promoting tissue repair, fat metabolism, and various other essential functions.[206] This phase serves as a sanctuary for your body, allowing it to heal and recover from the daily wear and tear.

Rapid Eye Movement (REM)

Rapid Eye Movement (REM) sleep is essential for your brain's growth, repair, and overall health. During REM, your brain transforms into a theater of dreams featuring vibrant, humorous, terrifying, and exciting experiences. These dreams help your brain process thoughts and emotions, consolidating information into memories.[207] REM constitutes 20-25% of your total sleep time, with some seasonal variations. Individuals experience approximately 16% more REM sleep in winter than in mid-summer.[208]

In REM sleep, your brain is "bathed" in cerebrospinal fluid, which aids in removing toxins and promotes neurogenesis – the growth of new brain cells.[209] Chronic sleep deprivation can impair your body's ability to generate new brain cells, leading to cognitive deficits.

An intriguing aspect of REM sleep relates to sexual arousal: penile erections and clitoral swelling occur during this phase. For men, the absence of morning erections may signal low testosterone levels or insufficient REM sleep. It's worth noting, particularly for men aged 40 and above, that improving sleep quality and consistency may alleviate concerns about libido or the absence of morning erections, potentially reducing the need for testosterone boosters or hormone therapy.[210]

Spending adequate time in each sleep phase bolsters your body's circadian rhythm, a 24-hour cycle that governs hormone and neurotransmitter production. Sufficient, high-quality sleep facilitates the following hormonal secretions:

1. Growth Hormone: The highest secretion within the 24-hour cycle occurs during deep sleep, with additional pulses released during each subsequent deep sleep cycle.[211]
2. Thyroid Stimulating Hormone (TSH): Peaks in the evening and decreases throughout the night, suggesting that thyroid hormones (T3 & T4) rise as the night progresses.[212]
3. Testosterone: In men, secretion is lowest around 8 pm and peaks around 8 am, so early morning blood tests are recommended for accurate assessment.[213]
4. Melatonin: Levels begin to rise at bedtime and peak between 3 am and 5 am.[214]
5. Leptin: Increases to suppress appetite.[215]
6. Cortisol, Epinephrine, Norepinephrine: Stress hormones

and neurotransmitters decrease during sleep and rise as morning approaches, preparing your body to wake up.[216]

Now that you know how important sleep is and what it means to get *enough quality* sleep, in the next chapter, we'll look at how you can get more quality sleep each night.

12

Sleep Hygiene

Now that you know how crucial *quality* sleep is for your long-term health, you might wonder, "How can I improve my sleep quality and quantity?" The following are the places to start.

Limit or Eliminate Alcohol

Drinking alcohol disrupts sleep patterns and decreases sleep quality, even when consumed in moderation.

One study found that alcohol consumption decreased sleep quality and increased sleep fragmentation, resulting in less restorative sleep.[217] Another study found that alcohol consumption before bed increased the occurrence of breathing disturbances during sleep, such as sleep apnea and snoring.[218] Alcohol consumption can also lead to decreased REM sleep.[219]

Go to Sleep at a Consistent Time

For your circadian rhythm to have a rhythm, you must go to sleep at a consistent time each night.[220] That might mean going to bed earlier than you're used to, especially if you don't usually go right to sleep after bed. Melatonin secretion initiates the process of putting you to sleep. But if you keep yourself up with artificial lights, digital screens, and stimulants, eventually, your body stops producing melatonin like it's supposed to. Then, when you want to sleep on schedule, you won't be able to.

If you have a hard time falling asleep, read a book. Just avoid books that make your mind start spinning, like books on politics or business. Read fiction instead. Your brain enters a state while reading similar to when you sleep, which is probably why so many people find it easy to fall asleep after reading a few pages but can stay awake for hours while watching a movie in bed.

Turn Down the Temperature

The ideal temperature at night is 67–69° Fahrenheit. Because your body doesn't regulate temperature as well while you're sleeping, you'll wake up if you get too hot.[221] It *is* possible to go too low with the temperature, though. Doing so reduces REM sleep. This is a survival mechanism common among mammals. You wouldn't want to be dead to the world because you're in a dream while your body freezes to death.[222]

Stop Eating a Few Hours Before Bedtime

It takes a few hours after a meal for blood sugar to return to normal, which then brings insulin levels back down. If insulin is elevated, it can blunt growth hormone secretion, which compromises the benefits of deep sleep.

Block Blue Light

Natural light contains some blue light, but we don't *naturally* get blue light after dark. Blue light exposure after dark interferes with melatonin secretion.[223] Many smartphones and laptops now have settings that allow you to shut off the blue light at night. I'd recommend wearing a pair of blue-light-blocking glasses after dark to minimize your eyes' exposure to blue light, as well. For that matter, keep your room as dark as possible, eliminating all potential light sources.

Deal With Stress

How does stress impact sleep? Holding onto stress and the accompanying emotions cause a cascade of hormones and neurotransmitters that keep you from sleeping well and further disrupt your metabolism.[224]

Consider Trying Sleep-Supporting Supplements

The following are some of the best supplements for supporting sleep. However, they're not the only supplements. As a reminder, always check with your healthcare practitioner before introducing supplements into your nutrition and lifestyle program, especially if you take medications or are being treated for a disease.

Magnesium L-Threonate

Magnesium L-threonate is a highly bioavailable form of magnesium that has been shown to support sleep by modulating neurotransmitters and hormones involved in the sleep-wake cycle.[225] As a critical cofactor in over 300 enzymatic reactions, magnesium plays a crucial role in regulating GABA, a neurotransmitter that promotes relaxation and sleep.[226] Studies have shown that magnesium L-threonate can effectively cross the blood-brain barrier, thus increasing brain magnesium levels and promoting synaptic plasticity, the ability of neurons to communicate with one another. Furthermore, magnesium supplementation has been linked to improving sleep quality, especially in individuals with insomnia.[227]

Essential Oils

Essential oils have been used for centuries to support sleep due to their soothing and calming properties. They are believed to impact the nervous system by influencing the limbic system, which plays a key role in regulating emotions and the sleep-wake cycle.[228] Aromatherapy, the practice of using essential oils for therapeutic purposes, has been shown to promote relaxation and improve sleep quality.[229] Lavender oil is the most well-known and extensively studied essential oil for sleep support, with research indicating its efficacy in reducing anxiety and promoting restful sleep.[230] Other effective essential oils for sleep include chamomile, bergamot, and ylang-ylang,

which exhibit sedative and anxiolytic (anxiety-reducing) properties.[231]

Several other oils can support sleep by promoting relaxation,
reducing stress, and improving overall sleep quality. Some
of these oils include clary sage, which has been found to
exhibit stress-reducing properties;[232] cedarwood, known for
its calming and grounding effects;[233] and valerian, which has
been traditionally used for its sedative and sleep-enhancing
properties.[234]

Relora®

Relora is a natural supplement derived from the extracts of two
plant species, *Magnolia officinalis* and *Phellodendron amurense*,
that is reported to support healthy sleep patterns. The primary
mechanism by which Relora is believed to promote sleep is
through its anxiolytic and stress-reducing properties, which
are attributed to its bioactive compounds, such as honokiol and
berberine.[235] These compounds have been shown to modulate
the activity of the central nervous system by interacting with
GABA receptors, thereby reducing stress and anxiety levels.[236]
As a result, Relora may facilitate better sleep quality by alleviating stress-related sleep disturbances.[237]

PharmaGABA

PharmaGABA, a natural form of gamma-aminobutyric acid
(GABA), supports sleep by promoting relaxation and reducing
anxiety. GABA, a primary inhibitory neurotransmitter in the
central nervous system, plays a crucial role in regulating the
sleep-wake cycle by inhibiting excitatory neurotransmitters

and inducing calmness.[238] PharmaGABA, as a bioavailable supplement, increases GABA levels in the brain, allowing for enhanced relaxation and facilitating sleep onset.[239] Additionally, studies have shown that PharmaGABA administration before bedtime may improve sleep quality by increasing the duration of deep, restorative sleep stages, such as slow-wave sleep.[240]

5-Hydroxytryptophan

5-Hydroxytryptophan (5-HTP) is a naturally occurring amino acid and a precursor to the neurotransmitter serotonin, which plays a crucial role in regulating sleep.[241] 5-HTP is synthesized from the essential amino acid tryptophan and is further converted into serotonin in the brain. Serotonin, in turn, can be converted into melatonin, a hormone that regulates the sleep-wake cycle.[242] By increasing the availability of serotonin and subsequently melatonin, 5-HTP has been suggested to improve sleep quality and support sleep initiation.[243]

L-Theanine

L-theanine, an amino acid found predominantly in green tea (*Camellia sinensis*), has been shown to support sleep by promoting relaxation and improving sleep quality.[244,245] L-theanine is thought to exert its sleep-promoting effects by increasing the levels of gamma-aminobutyric acid (GABA), serotonin, and dopamine in the brain, neurotransmitters that play crucial roles in regulating sleep and mood.[246,247] Additionally, l-theanine has been found to reduce the latency of sleep onset and improve sleep efficiency, without causing daytime drowsiness or dependence.[248] These findings suggest that l-theanine supplementation may be a safe and effective natural sleep aid for individuals experiencing sleep disturbances.

Melatonin

Melatonin is a hormone produced by the pineal gland in the brain, which plays a crucial role in regulating sleep-wake cycles.[249] The synthesis and release of melatonin are influenced by the body's internal clock, known as the circadian rhythm, and environmental factors like light exposure.[250] When it gets dark, melatonin production increases, signaling the body that it is time to sleep. Conversely, exposure to light, particularly blue light, suppresses melatonin release, promoting wakefulness.[251] Studies have shown that melatonin supplements can treat insomnia and sleep disorders, especially in individuals with delayed sleep phase syndrome or jet lag.[252,253]

Melatonin's role in supporting sleep extends beyond its regulation of the sleep-wake cycle. Recent research has explored how melatonin interacts with other sleep-related processes and neurotransmitters, such as gamma-aminobutyric acid (GABA) and serotonin. Melatonin has been found to modulate GABAergic transmission, enhancing the inhibitory effects of GABA on neuronal activity, which may contribute to sleep initiation and maintenance.[254] Additionally, melatonin is synthesized from the amino acid tryptophan, which is a precursor to serotonin, another neurotransmitter involved in regulating sleep and mood.[255]

The efficacy of melatonin as a sleep aid varies across different populations, including children, adults, and the elderly. Melatonin has been found to be particularly effective in improving sleep quality and reducing sleep onset latency in children with neurodevelopmental disorders, such as autism spectrum disorder and attention deficit hyperactivity disorder (ADHD).[256] In elderly individuals, melatonin supplementation may help counteract age-related declines in melatonin production, improving sleep quality and reducing the risk of sleep disturbances.[257]

2555

2,555 – that's the minimum number of hours you should sleep each year as an adult. Just as a plane can veer miles off course by deviating only a degree or two, your health and fitness can deteriorate when you consistently sacrifice even a small amount of sleep night after night.

Falling short by just 30 minutes every night accumulates to 182.5 hours over a year—equivalent to more than an entire week of lost sleep. This sleep debt can wreak havoc on your mental and physical health, potentially resulting in significant muscle loss. The time you gain by staying up later will ultimately be squandered through poor health and, possibly, a shorter lifespan.

Invest in your future self rather than stealing from it. Prioritize sleep by going to bed earlier, and reap the benefits of a healthier, more vigorous life.

V

Living the 3 Pillars

*If it is important to you, you will find a way. If not,
you will find an excuse.*
– Anonymous

13

Becoming Nonnegotiable

As you've read about The 3 Pillars of Vigor, you may have noticed the overlapping health benefits of resistance training, high-protein diets, and adequate sleep. These three choices work synergistically to build muscle and maximize health.

Strength training initiates muscle growth, protein supplies the building blocks necessary for muscle development, and sleep fosters the hormonal environment that facilitates muscle growth.

You may have also observed the significant roles these three factors play in:

- Maintaining blood pressure, lipid levels, and cardiovascular health
- Supporting a robust immune system
- Enhancing cognitive function
- Reducing body fat and improving body composition
- Balancing sex and metabolic hormones
- Alleviating anxiety and depression

By now, you should understand the immense power these three simple habits hold for your current and future well-being, as well as for those who follow your example. The next step is to integrate these practices into your daily routine, not just temporarily, but for the rest of your life. Commit to these non-negotiable habits and watch as they transform your health and vitality.

Making the Pillars Work In Your Life

Each day, you make roughly 35,000 decisions. While that number may seem staggering, most of these choices aren't life-changing. However, some seemingly minor or inconsequential decisions can have a significant impact when repeated over time. Consistently making poor choices can lead you astray from the life you envision for your future self.

For instance, consider the following situations:

1. Your alarm sounds at 5:30 am. The bed is cozy, and the pillow is soft. It's dark and quiet outside. You're tempted by the prospect of another hour of sleep and rationalize that sleep is good for you. So, do you hit snooze and skip your workout, or do you get up and head to the gym?
2. After getting ready for the day, it's time for breakfast. You know that cooking eggs and bacon or making a low-carb protein shake is a healthier option, but the convenience of a bowl of cereal is tempting. Do you choose the quick fix, or do you prioritize your health and that of your family?
3. At work, a coworker brings in coffee and donuts for some-one's birthday. Although you recognize the unhealthy nature of the treat, the allure of free food and the special

occasion is strong. Do you indulge in the donuts or stick to just the coffee?

Situations like these arise daily. Relying solely on willpower can often lead you to choose immediate gratification over long-term benefits, resulting in guilt and disappointment.

Willpower and Decision Fatigue

Every day, you'll face temptations that go against your best interests. You might feel the urge to gossip, complain, or make choices that weaken your resolve. To overcome these challenges, you need willpower, right?

Willpower is the mental control exerted to accomplish something or resist impulses. It's the mental energy required to make the right choices and avoid the wrong ones. Many people believe that healthier individuals simply possess stronger willpower. That's rarely the case.

In their book, *Willpower: Rediscovering the Greatest Human Strength*, Roy Baumeister and John Tierney define decision fatigue as "the deteriorating quality of decisions made by an individual after a long session of decision-making."

As you make more decisions, your willpower weakens. Negotiating with yourself to make the best choices becomes increasingly tricky. This is why scheduling significant meetings at the end of the workday or making critical family decisions late at night can be detrimental.

Throughout the day, as you navigate various decisions related to family, work, finances, and fitness, the quality of your choices declines. An exhausting workday, followed by time spent choosing the perfect outfit for dinner, can significantly impair your ability to make wise selections from the restaurant menu. Similarly, if you opt to stay home, deciding on a meal can feel overwhelming, potentially leading to unhealthy choices like ordering pizza.

To combat decision fatigue and preserve your willpower, it's crucial to create routines and strategies that minimize the number of decisions you need to make daily, especially concerning your health and fitness goals.

How to Conserve Your Willpower

Each day, you begin with a specific amount of willpower. If you wake up tired from the previous day, your willpower reserves may not be fully recharged. Nevertheless, this doesn't excuse you from making good decisions – you are still accountable for each choice you make. To ensure you have enough willpower for the most important decisions, learning how to conserve it is essential.

Consider your willpower like a cell phone battery. When it's running low, and you don't have access to a charger, you'll use your phone sparingly and focus on the essentials. You might disable notifications, close background apps, and reduce screen brightness to conserve battery life. Similarly, you can adopt strategies to preserve your willpower for critical decisions:

1. Make fewer decisions: Simplify your life by establishing routines and habits that minimize the number of choices you need to make daily. For example, prepare your gym clothes the night before or make your meal for the next day, so that the next day you won't be tempted to eat something you shouldn't.

2. Turn certain decisions into non-negotiable activities: Prioritize essential health and fitness goals by making them non-negotiable aspects of your daily routine. Treat these activities like brushing your teeth or going to work – they are simply part of your day, and there's no need to debate whether to do them or not.

Make Fewer Decisions

If decisions deplete your willpower reserves, it makes sense to reduce the number of choices you need to make. With 35,000 decisions to make daily, where do you start? Focus on the conscious decisions that tend to cause decision fatigue and drain your willpower.

Steve Jobs was known for wearing the same outfit every day. It wasn't the same shirt and pair of jeans; he had multiple pairs. This approach eliminated one of the most common early-morning decisions people face: "What should I wear today?" Simple, right?

Consider streamlining your meal choices as well. You could have a few different lunches throughout the week, consistent from one week to the next, to avoid the question, "What should I eat for lunch?" Similarly, have a few go-to dinner options to minimize decision-making around "What's for dinner?"

If breakfast is a challenge, clear out your pantry and decide on a few healthy options like eggs and bacon, or protein shakes, that align with your nutritional goals. Remove everything else, and you'll eliminate many decisions while also improving your breakfast choices.

What's good for you is also beneficial for the rest of your family. Dispose of unhealthy options like breakfast cereal,

cereal bars, frozen waffles, and other junk food. If these items aren't in the house, you won't need to decide whether or not to eat them. By removing them, you eliminate the decision-making process and conserve your willpower for more important choices.

Make Frequent Decisions Nonnegotiable

Years ago, my wife, Vanessa, and I developed a concept for our network marketing team called a non-negotiable task list. We discovered that a minimal number of simple activities if practiced consistently, could all but guarantee someone's success in their business.

We called it the Nonnegotiable Diamond in the Making Task List because reaching the rank of Diamond and above leads to a lucrative and exciting business and lifestyle.

The idea remains the same whether you're building a successful business, a healthy body, or an educated and critically-thinking mind. To achieve success, you must consistently perform a few crucial activities.

I encourage you to make the following nonnegotiable:

1. Ensure each meal is high in protein
2. Strength train four days per week
3. Sleep at least seven hours each night

If you've never considered your decisions this way, you might be tempted to turn even more decisions into non-negotiables. However, I caution you against doing so. Begin with as few decisions as possible—the ones that will significantly impact the area of your life you're focusing on. Master consistency with these first, and then add others later. In terms of your health, please start with the three we've been discussing throughout this book.

Be Nonnegotiable But Flexible

Non-negotiables are not negotiable. You have to get them done. Once you've made the decisions, consuming enough protein and getting enough sleep should be relatively easy. However, what happens when your schedule changes or you go on vacation? How do you manage your workouts? You adapt your workout schedule.

As an example, while writing this section, Vanessa and I were on a ski vacation with our grandson, Asher. We left on Monday and returned on Friday. I adjusted my usual Monday, Tuesday, Thursday, Friday workout schedule for that week to Sunday, Monday (before we left), Friday (after we got home), and Saturday. I made this adjustment because I knew that working out while skiing so much would compromise my skiing performance. For most other vacations or trips we take, we stick to our normal workout routine. We choose hotels with adequate gyms or locations near gyms that we can use.

The point is that when strength training is nonnegotiable, it means you'll do what it takes to get it done, even if it requires flexibility and adaptation.

How to Make It Easier to Stick to Your Non-negotiables

Share Your Non-Negotiable Activities with Your Family and Significant Other

Your non-negotiables will sometimes inconvenience others, just as their non-negotiables inconvenience you. Talk to your family about how important this is for you so they understand why you need to be steadfast about the 3 Pillars.

Accept Accountability

If you expect your family to adjust to your nonnegotiables, you need to allow them to call you out if you're not following through. Seek accountability from your family, or if necessary, find it from a friend or workout partner.

An accountability partner isn't someone who makes you feel good about falling short or tolerates your excuses. They politely call you out on your inconsistencies. Too often, when we fail to follow our plan, we want someone to comfort us and tell us it's okay. We seek solace. After a while, we get comfortable with our failure, knowing that others will make us feel better.

You must break the cycle.

You have to get comfortable with the discomfort of someone else calling you out. Alternatively, commit to your plan and execute it, so you won't have to experience discomfort.

Eliminate Your Excuses

This might be difficult to accept, but almost any reason you can come up with for not strength training, eating a high-protein diet, or getting enough sleep is an excuse (mothers with babies are an exception regarding sleep debt).

How can you tell the difference between an excuse and a reason? Ask a three-word question: "Was it impossible?"

"You said you couldn't work out yesterday because you had company over. Was it impossible to work out for an hour out of the entire day?" "You said that the only food they served at our work lunch was sandwiches. Was it impossible to eat more protein (like having backup protein bars in your desk drawer)?" "You said you had a hectic week last week. Was it impossible to have gotten in two workouts during the week and two on the weekend?"

More often than not, what we're saying is that it was inconvenient, not impossible. If inconvenience stops you, it's an excuse. If it was impossible, it was a valid reason. You don't miss nonnegotiables because of inconvenience.

14

Dealing With Obstacles

Be Consistent

I've met many people who complained that their 12-week fitness program didn't work. While there are plenty of lousy programs out there, sold by people with minimal knowledge and even less experience, the more common problem is that those people expected to undo a lifetime of poor choices in three months' time. And often, in those three months, they'd admit that they didn't even follow their program consistently.

I've been strength training for 29 years, and during that time, the most I've ever missed is two weeks of training in a calendar year. Most years, I don't miss a week. Even last year, when I broke my neck, I missed less than a week. I estimate I've completed 5800 workouts. I've also been consistent with eating a high-protein diet for most of that time, and guarding my sleep against intruders and intrusions. I've *chosen* consistency.

That doesn't mean every workout was awesome, or I didn't eat absolute junk on top of the protein on occasion. I have missed some sleep now and then. But I've been *consistent*, and you need to be as well. Whether you're 39 or 93; consistency is crucial to living a healthy, fit, and long life.

Adjusting for Age

Though The 3 Pillars of Vigor work for people of all ages, older adults might need to make some adjustments.

As we age, our bodies become less efficient at processing and utilizing the nutrients needed for muscle growth and maintenance. This phenomenon, known as anabolic resistance, is a significant contributing factor to the loss of muscle mass and function in older adults.[258] The main factors contributing to anabolic resistance include reduced muscle protein synthesis in response to protein intake, decreased physical activity, and changes in hormonal levels.[259]

Basically, older adults don't respond to the same amount of protein or frequency of training as they did when they were younger. They need to eat more protein and eat it more often to stimulate muscle growth. To make things more challenging, appetite declines with age as well. Older adults must make a concerted effort to eat high-protein meals frequently throughout the day or at least consume high-protein supplements like bars or shakes. Branched-chain amino acid supplements between meals can also support the maintenance of muscle. They're also less filling, so they may be easier to use for older adults with reduced appetites.

Regarding resistance training, they may need to strength train more often, like five or six days per week instead of the standard three or four. Of course, they'd do fewer exercises with a higher frequency to avoid training more than they can recover from.

Finally, older adults often deal with poor sleep, partly because they don't secrete melatonin either. To protect their brains and bodies, it's essential to get to bed at a consistent time, and even to take a mid-afternoon nap whenever possible.

Dealing with Injuries

I often tell my clients, "You'll frequently feel sore, occasionally get hurt, and once in a while, get injured. Such is the nature of an active adult."

More often than not, people turn their injury into an excuse not to exercise when they should really use their injury as a reason to exercise. In 2008, I ruptured my left Achilles tendon while sprinting. I had it reattached and returned to the gym two days after surgery, training my uninjured right leg and my upper body. In 2013, I ruptured my left distal biceps tendon doing deadlifts. I worked out the next two days, then had surgery, and got back in the gym two days after that, training my uninjured right arm and my lower body. In the summer of 2022, I rode my mountain bike off a bridge, which threw me headfirst into the ground, fracturing two cervical vertebrae and causing significant spinal cord damage. I had an emergency surgery that day and left the hospital three days later. Two days after that, wearing a neck collar and with dysfunctional hands and severe upper body paralysis, I got back into the gym and started training what I could. Not surprisingly, in every case, I recovered in half the time the surgeons said it would take. Resistance training, a high-protein diet, and at least seven hours of sleep are nonnegotiable, especially when recovering from an injury, not just when you're healthy and injury-free.

15

Beyond the 3 Pillars

You've been consistent with The 3 Pillars. You see results, and you have enough margin in your schedule that you'd like to do more to improve your health. What's next?

I was hesitant about including this chapter. I don't want someone to believe they can skip over The 3 Pillars and start here instead, convincing themselves that *something is better than nothing.* I know many fitness professionals who tell their clients and followers such things. They want to appeal to everyone, so they tell people to do whatever feels good for them. But that's a temptation we must overcome...doing what feels good. It's what's gotten us into this unhealthy predicament to begin with.

However, I know that some people will already be consistent with The 3 Pillars. I'll recommend a few more things you could *add to* The 3 Pillars of Vigor.

Take The Foundational 5

Five supplements stand out as the most valuable for the majority of people. I call them The Foundational Five. If you're being treated for a medical condition or taking a prescription, always consult your doctor before introducing new supplements to your nutrition program.

High-Quality Multivitamin

Studies have shown that taking a high-quality multivitamin may help reduce the risk of chronic diseases like heart disease, cancer, and diabetes.[260] Multivitamin and mineral supplements can help fill nutritional gaps in the diet,[261] providing essential vitamins and minerals such as vitamin C, vitamin D, vitamin E, and calcium, among others.

Vitamins and minerals are critical in immune function, cognitive function, and brain health. For example, vitamin C is a potent antioxidant that helps protect the body against damage from free radicals. These compounds accelerate the aging process and may contribute to cancer production. They can also cause chronic inflammation and weaken the immune system. Vitamin B12 is essential for maintaining healthy nerve cells and cognitive function. Folate, another B vitamin, is essential for brain function and may help reduce the risk of age-related cognitive decline.[262]

As we age, our bodies may become less efficient at absorbing and utilizing nutrients from food. A high-quality multivitamin can help bridge this gap by providing essential nutrients that support healthy aging. For example, vitamin D is vital for maintaining bone health, while vitamins E and C are antioxidants that help protect against cellular damage and oxidative stress.

Fish Oil

Omega-3 fatty acids may help reduce triglyceride levels and lower the risk of heart disease.[263] These fatty acids may also help reduce inflammation in the body, which can contribute to the development of heart disease. In addition to heart health benefits, fish oil supplements may help reduce joint pain and stiffness in people with rheumatoid arthritis.[264] Omega-3 fatty acids have anti-inflammatory properties that can help reduce inflammation and swelling, improving overall joint health.

Omega-3 fatty acids are also crucial for brain function and may help improve mental health. Studies have shown that supplementing with fish oil can help improve both mood and cognitive function, and reduce symptoms of depression and anxiety.[265] Furthermore, omega-3 fatty acids are essential for maintaining eye health. Studies have shown that supplementing with fish oil may help reduce the risk of age-related macular degeneration (AMD) and dry eye syndrome.[266] Finally, some studies suggest that omega-3 fatty acids may help reduce the risk of certain types of cancer, including breast, colon, and prostate cancer.[267]

Magnesium

Magnesium deficiency is one of the top two micronutrient deficiencies. Due to its size, it's challenging to fit a full dose of magnesium into a multivitamin formulation, so you'll probably need to take it as a separate supplement.

Magnesium is an essential mineral that is important in many

bodily functions. Supplementing with magnesium may offer several potential health benefits, including improved bone health by regulating the body's calcium and vitamin D levels.[268] Magnesium may also help reduce the risk of developing type 2 diabetes by improving insulin sensitivity and regulating blood sugar levels.[269] Furthermore, magnesium may help improve sleep quality and duration, particularly in older adults.[270] It helps regulate the body's melatonin levels, a hormone that regulates sleep. Studies have also shown magnesium may help reduce the frequency and severity of migraines,[271] likely due to its ability to relax blood vessels and reduce inflammation. Finally, magnesium may help reduce symptoms of anxiety and depression by regulating neurotransmitters in the brain, including serotonin, which is vital for mood regulation.[272]

Vitamin D

Vitamin D is actually a prohormone, or hormone precursor, that plays a vital role in many bodily functions. However, more than half of the world's population is deficient in vitamin D, and as many as four out of five people in the United States may have below-optimal levels.[273] Low blood levels of vitamin D increase the risk factors for diabetes, arthritis, dementia, and bone loss. It may also increase the risk of viral infections such as the flu.[274]

Fortunately, the most common micronutrient deficiency in the world is easily preventable. High-quality supplements are inexpensive, and if you live in the right latitude, you can get a healthy dose from moderate mid-day sun exposure. Vitamin D is consumed in two forms: ergocalciferol (D2) and cholecalciferol (D3). Vitamin D3 is far superior.

Even if you consume fortified foods like orange juice or milk, you may still fall short of optimal cholecalciferol intake. The best food sources of cholecalciferol include fatty fish, beef liver, and cod liver oil.[275] Also, most multivitamins err on the side of too little rather than too much. So, like magnesium, you'll likely need a separate vitamin D supplement.

Vitamin D deficiency is associated with many adverse health outcomes, including a higher risk of respiratory tract infections, cardiovascular disease, and autoimmune diseases. A study showed that supplementing with 2000 IU of cholecalciferol lessens cold and flu symptoms.[276] Another study found that raising vitamin D levels in those with insulin resistance reduces the symptoms of insulin resistance, which can lead to type 2 diabetes.[277] Low vitamin D levels increase the risk of developing metabolic syndrome by 52%.

Vitamin D also plays a role in supporting bone health by mediating calcium absorption. Taking tons of calcium is pointless without sufficient magnesium and vitamins K and D.[278] Moreover, vitamin D may also be beneficial for cognitive function during pregnancy. A study published in *The Journal of Nutrition* showed that mothers with higher vitamin D levels during pregnancy had children with higher IQs when measured at 4-6 years old.[279]

Probiotics or Digestive Enzymes

Depending on the individual, I could go either way with the fifth of the Foundational 5. I often lean towards digestive enzymes to maximize digestion and absorption of the foods you eat. Still, there's definitely a valid argument for making probiotics the fifth of the five. I'll provide an overview of the benefits of each here for you.

Probiotics

Probiotics can help to prevent and treat various diseases, including antibiotic-associated diarrhea, irritable bowel syndrome, and inflammatory bowel disease.[280]

Probiotics improve digestive health by breaking down food and producing enzymes the human body cannot produce. They can also help to reduce inflammation in the gut and improve the gut barrier function, which is critical for preventing harmful substances from entering the bloodstream. Additionally, probiotics can help to alleviate symptoms of lactose intolerance and increase the bioavailability of certain nutrients, such as calcium, iron, and magnesium.[281]

Probiotics have also been shown to enhance immune function by increasing the production of cytokines, which are proteins that regulate the immune system. They also help maintain a healthy balance of gut bacteria, which is essential for optimal immune function. Studies have shown that consuming probiotics can reduce the risk and duration of respiratory infections, urinary tract infections, and other infections.

Finally, probiotics may also have a positive impact on mental health. Research has shown that the gut and the brain are connected, and a healthy gut microbiome may help to reduce symptoms of anxiety, depression, and stress. Probiotics have been shown to reduce symptoms of depression and anxiety in several clinical trials.[282]

Digestive Enzymes

Digestive enzymes have been shown to offer several health benefits. They can help improve digestion, alleviate symptoms of digestive disorders, and promote nutrient absorption. A study on subjects with digestive enzyme insufficiency found that a supplement containing proteases, amylases, and lipases improved digestion and reduced symptoms such as bloating, gas, and abdominal pain. Furthermore, enzyme supplementation has been found to alleviate symptoms of irritable bowel syndrome (IBS) and inflammatory bowel disease (IBD).[283]

Additionally, digestive enzymes can help improve nutrient absorption. Nutrient absorption may be compromised when the body cannot break down food properly. This can lead to nutrient deficiencies, even in individuals with a healthy diet. Digestive enzymes can help break down food and improve nutrient absorption, potentially improving overall health and well-being.[284]

Moreover, proteolytic (protein-digesting) enzymes have been found to have anti-inflammatory effects, which may offer additional health benefits. A study conducted on patients with osteoarthritis found that supplementation with proteolytic enzymes reduced inflammation and improved joint function.[285] Similarly, proteolytic enzymes have been found to reduce inflammation and swelling in athletes following strenuous exercise.[286]

Walk and Move Frequently

Sitting for long periods is associated with various adverse health outcomes, including obesity, type 2 diabetes, cardiovascular disease, and premature mortality. Moving frequently throughout the day, on the other hand, has been linked to improved cardiovascular health, metabolic function, and brain function, as well as reduced risk of chronic disease and premature death.[287,288,289]

Research shows that breaking up periods of prolonged sitting with short bouts of light-intensity physical activity, such as standing or walking, can improve blood glucose and insulin levels, decrease blood pressure, and improve lipid profiles.[290,291,292] Even short breaks of light-intensity activity can make a difference. One study found that taking a 2-minute walk every 30 minutes was more effective at reducing post-meal glucose levels than a 30-minute walk once daily.[293]

Frequent movement throughout the day can also have positive effects on brain function. Studies show that physical activity can improve cognitive function, including attention, working memory, and decision-making.[294,295,296] Additionally, light-intensity activity, such as standing, can improve mood and reduce stress.[297,298]

The benefits of frequent movement throughout the day are not limited to physical and cognitive health. In a study of office workers, those who had sit-stand workstations reported improved job performance, decreased fatigue, and reduced musculoskeletal discomfort compared to those who had traditional seated workstations.[299] Additionally, frequent movement throughout the day can improve sleep quality and duration, which is important for overall health and well-being.

Overall, it's clear that frequent movement throughout the day is important for overall health and well-being. Incorporating short bouts of light-intensity physical activity, such as standing, walking, or stretching, into your daily routine can positively impact physical and cognitive health, job performance, and sleep quality. You could even go for a long walk or do some zone 2, or low-intensity, fat-burning cardio if you wish. But do it to be active rather than thinking you need to add another workout to your schedule.

Eat Meals, Not Snacks

For much of my 20 years as a fitness professional, conventional nutrition advice said that people are better off eating four, five, or even six times per day than eating one, two, or three times per day. Early in my career, I encouraged clients to eat every few hours, meaning they snacked multiple times each day.

In recent years, research has emerged showing that snacking may actually be detrimental to your health and weight management. My personal experience and the results coming from my clients attest to that.

I recommend avoiding snacks for multiple reasons. Some relate to your behavior. Others relate to your hormones and metabolism.

Eating Often Conditions You to Eat Often

If you intend to eat five times daily, you'll have to eat every three to four hours. You'll have to think about your next meal not long after your current meal. It doesn't take much for your thoughts about eating to become an obsession. If you eat less often, you'll think about eating less often because you have to plan to eat less often.

Snack foods are some of the most addicting foods on the planet. Loaded with artificial flavors and rich in fat and carbohydrates, they satisfy more than cravings. They give you a temporary high followed by hedonic hunger.

Of course, most snack food companies don't want you to know this. The snack food industry generates more than $45 billion per year.

Research shows that although many nutrition and fitness professionals advocate eating small, frequent meals, such practices offer no benefits in metabolism or appetite and are more likely to have the opposite effect of stimulating hunger and reducing satiety.[300]

Increased Carbohydrate Consumption

Aside from a personal trainer who weighs, measures, and packs every meal and snack, most people who eat snacks or eat more than three meals per day eat significantly more carbohydrates than those who eat just two or three meals daily.

Once your carbohydrate stores are full, you convert those extra carbohydrates to triglycerides and body fat while keeping blood sugar and insulin levels higher than healthy levels for more of your day.

Suppressed Growth Hormone

It takes about three hours to digest and absorb a meal and for your blood sugar and insulin levels to return to normal. Growth hormone levels start to rise about that time, increasing fat metabolism and enhancing tissue growth and repair.

Those who eat within a few hours of a previous meal miss out on this growth hormone secretion. Imagine the impact of getting a couple of extra natural doses of growth hormone each day compared to the person who eats all day long and only experiences an increase in growth hormone during sleep (if they get good quality sleep).

Leptin and ghrelin (your hunger hormones) secretion may also get sabotaged by eating too often. In essence, you train yourself to be in constant hunger or cravings.

In a study of more than 50,000 Seventh-day Adventists, researchers examined whether eating fewer meals each day led to better body composition. They found that the more meals people eat, the more they weigh.[301] The study authors believed lower meal frequency led to less oxidative stress, improved satiety, and better circadian rhythm, impacting sleep quality and hunger-related and sex hormone balance.

Two or Three Square Meals Per Day

It wasn't until recently that humans could eat all day long. Throughout history, we ate one or two meals, sometimes three. But, with patience and persistence, you can wean yourself off the cravings and get back to eating two or three square meals per day. Here's how.

Eat High-Protein

Before I have clients eat fewer meals, I first have them eat more protein, beginning with their first meal. If you've made it this far, you already do that since a high-protein diet is one of The

3 Pillars of Vigor.

After clients get consistent with eating high-protein at all meals and snacks, I have them remove one meal or snack at a time. Over time, we work our way down to two or three meals per day.

Eat at Consistent Times

While eating fewer meals each day provides numerous health benefits, there's one caveat: Eat your meals at consistent times.

Our bodies operate with a circadian rhythm. Though our sleep patterns affect circadian rhythm, so does our eating pattern. People who eat only two or three meals daily and eat them at inconsistent times tend to be heavier and less healthy. Conversely, eating only two or three meals per day at *consistent* times leads to better health and body composition.[302] For example, perhaps you've eaten a meal much later than usual, and the next morning you feel unusually hungry. Your late-night meal might have disrupted your ghrelin and leptin levels, the hormones that affect hunger and satiety.

Get Active Instead of Eating

Find something else to do if you've developed a snacking pattern at a specific time. Do lawn work, go to the gym, walk through a park, or find another activity that takes your mind off eating. If you have a habit of eating while working, scrolling through social media, or doing something else, you need to find something different to do. *Hoping* not to eat while doing the same things you've done before *while* eating, is a recipe for failure.

Eat Dessert with Dinner

If you tend to eat a snack late at night, you probably don't need to give up the snack. You just need to eat it as part of dinner.

As I often tell my clients, your meal is over when you leave the table, so eat what you want while you're sitting at it. Provided you ate a high-protein dinner, if you're going to eat something sweet, you're better off eating it right after your meal as part of your meal than eating it later in the evening as a "snack."

16

Concluding Thoughts

The power of social influence cannot be underestimated, especially regarding our choices related to our health and well-being. The people we surround ourselves with can tremendously impact our lifestyle, from the activities we engage in to the foods we eat. Studies have demonstrated that our social networks significantly influence our health behaviors, reinforcing the importance of choosing our company wisely.

One study found that obesity can be socially contagious.[303] When a person becomes obese, their friends are 57% more likely to become obese as well. This ripple effect spreads through our social networks, underlining the importance of surrounding ourselves with individuals who prioritize a healthy lifestyle. Spending time with health-conscious friends makes us more likely to adopt their habits and benefit from a healthier lifestyle.

In addition to influencing our eating habits, our social circles also influence our physical activity levels. A study by the University of Pennsylvania demonstrated that social influence can be an effective motivator for exercise.[304] Participants who exercised with friends reported greater enjoyment and more motivation to engage in physical activities than those who exercised alone. This underscores the value of selecting active friends who share our commitment to fitness.

Furthermore, the support we receive from our social networks can significantly impact our mental health. Strong social connections have been shown to reduce the risk of depression, anxiety, and other mental health issues.[305] By fostering relationships with individuals who share our values and goals, we can create an environment that is conducive to emotional well-being.

In conclusion, the people we surround ourselves with play a vital role in shaping our choices, especially those related to our health. By consciously selecting friends who prioritize a healthy lifestyle, we can reap the benefits of their influence in our lives. Ultimately, the power of social connections can be harnessed to help us achieve our health and fitness goals and lead a more fulfilling life.

Do Not Grow Soft

Long ago, Seneca said, "It is a shame for a man to grow old without seeing the beauty and strength of which his body is capable." In a selfie-filled, narcissistic culture, it's easy to take those words at face value and think of a fit body as an aesthetic thing. I've always seen it differently. I view the process of building and maintaining a strong, fit body—one that embraces the difficult task of lifting weights, choosing protein-rich foods over carb and fat-filled junk, and putting the phone and social media away to get a good night's sleep—as an opportunity to add beauty, strength, and value to the world in which that body resides. There's no question that we offer the most value to the world when our bodies and minds work as well as possible. When we're strong, fit, resilient, healthy, and energetic.

I don't want to grow soft because I know I'll function at a fraction of my abilities. But more importantly, at a fraction of my abilities, I won't be able to contribute as effectively to my family, nor will I be able to set an example for the next generations in my family, such as for our grandson.

If you feel the same, I urge you to implement The 3 Pillars of Vigor in your own life and then pass them along to those who marvel at the vigorous person you have become. Don't grow soft.

Notes

INTRODUCTION

1   Plato. (2003). The Republic (B. Jowett, Trans.). Dover Publications.

2   Kaeuper, R. W. (1999). Chivalry and violence in medieval Europe. Oxford University Press.

3   Gouwens, K. (2006). The Renaissance man and his children: Humanism and Aristotelianism in Renaissance Italy. Renaissance Quarterly, 59(2), 305-353.

4   Kasson, J. F. (2001). Houdini, Tarzan, and the perfect man: The white male body and the challenge of modernity in America. Hill and Wang.

5   Merriam-Webster. (n.d.). Vigor. In Merriam-Webster.com dictionary. Retrieved March 16, 2023, from https://www.merriam-webster.com/dictionary/vigor

MUSCLE MASS: HEALTH, FITNESS, AND LONGEVITY.

6   MacIntosh, B. R., Gardiner, P. F., & McComas, A. J. (2006). Skeletal muscle: Form and function. Human Kinetics.

7   Sanders, K M. "Regulation of smooth muscle excitation and contraction." *Neurogastroenterology and motility : the official journal of the European Gastrointestinal Motility Society* vol. 20 Suppl 1,Suppl 1 (2008): 39-53. doi:10.1111/j.1365-2982.2008.01108.x

8   Katz, A. M. (2006). Physiology of the heart. Lippincott Williams & Wilkins.

9   Pette, D., & Staron, R. S. (2001). Transitions of muscle fiber phenotypic profiles. Histochemistry and cell biology, 115(5), 359-372.

10 Komi, P. V., Viitasalo, J. H., Rauramaa, R., & Vihko, V. (1980). Effect of isometric strength training on mechanical, electrical, and metabolic aspects of muscle function. European Journal of Applied Physiology and Occupational Physiology, 40(1), 45-55.

11 Rayment, I et al. "Structure of the actin-myosin complex and its implications for muscle contraction." *Science (New York, N.Y.)* vol. 261,5117 (1993): 58-65. doi:10.1126/science.8316858

12   Burd, N. A., Andrews, R. J., West, D. W., Little, J. P., Cochran, A. J., Hector, A. J., ... & Phillips, S. M. (2012). Muscle time under tension during resistance exercise stimulates differential muscle protein sub-fractional synthetic responses in men. The Journal of Physiology, 590(2), 351-362.

13   Schoenfeld, B. J. (2013). Potential mechanisms for a role of metabolic stress in hypertrophic adaptations to resistance training. Sports Medicine, 43(3), 179-194.

14   Schoenfeld, B. J. (2012). Does exercise-induced muscle damage play a role in skeletal muscle hypertrophy? Journal of Strength and Conditioning Research, 26(5), 1441-1453.

15   Damas, F., Phillips, S. M., Libardi, C. A., Vechin, F. C., Lixandrão, M. E., Jannig, P. R., ... & Ugrinowitsch, C. (2016). Resistance training-induced changes in integrated myofibrillar protein synthesis are related to hypertrophy only after attenuation of muscle damage. The Journal of Physiology, 594(18), 5209-5222.

16   Loenneke, J. P., Wilson, J. M., Marín, P. J., Zourdos, M. C., & Bemben, M. G. (2012). Low-intensity blood flow restriction training: a meta-analysis. European Journal of Applied Physiology, 112(5), 1849-1859. DOI: **https://d oi.org/10.1007/s00421-011-2167-x**

17   Kon, M., Ohiwa, N., Honda, A., Matsubayashi, T., Ikeda, T., Akimoto, T., Suzuki, Y., Hirano, Y., & Russell, A. P. (2014). Effects of systemic hypoxia on human muscular adaptations to resistance exercise training. Physiological Reports, 2(6), e12033. DOI: **https://doi.org/10.14814/phy2.12033**

18   Fry, A. C. (2004). The role of resistance exercise intensity on muscle fibre adaptations. Sports Medicine, 34(10), 663-679.

19   Keller K, Engelhardt M. Strength and muscle mass loss with aging process. Age and strength loss. Muscles Ligaments Tendons J. 2014 Feb 24;3(4):346-50. PMID: 24596700; PMCID: PMC3940510.

20   Wolfe RR. The underappreciated role of muscle in health and disease. Am J Clin Nutr. 2006 Sep;84(3):475-82. doi: 10.1093/ajcn/84.3.475. PMID: 16960159.

21   Wolfe RR. The underappreciated role of muscle in health and disease. Am J Clin Nutr. 2006 Sep;84(3):475-82. doi: 10.1093/ajcn/84.3.475. PMID: 16960159.

22   Srikanthan, P., & Karlamangla, A. S. (2014). Muscle mass index as a predictor of longevity in older adults. The American Journal of Medicine, 127(6), 547-553.

23 Kim, T. N., Park, M. S., Yang, S. J., Yoo, H. J., Kang, H. J., Song, W., ... & Lee, S. K. (2013). Prevalence and determinant factors of insulin resistance in non-diabetic Korean women: results from the Korea National Health and Nutrition Examination Survey, 2008-2010. PloS one, 8(5), e66119.

24 Goodpaster, B. H., Park, S. W., Harris, T. B., Kritchevsky, S. B., Nevitt, M., Schwartz, A. V., ... & Newman, A. B. (2006). The loss of skeletal muscle mass and strength in older adults: the health, aging and body composition study. Journal of gerontology: Medical Sciences, 61(10), 1059-1064.

25 James SL, Lucchesi LR, Bisignano C, Castle CD, Dingels ZV, Fox JT, Hamilton EB, Henry NJ, Krohn KJ, Liu Z, McCracken D, Nixon MR, Roberts NLS, Sylte DO, Adsuar JC, Arora A, Briggs AM, Collado-Mateo D, Cooper C, Dandona L, Dandona R, Ellingsen CL, Fereshtehnejad SM, Gill TK, Haagsma JA, Hendrie D, Jürisson M, Kumar GA, Lopez AD, Miazgowski T, Miller TR, Mini GK, Mirrakhimov EM, Mohamadi E, Olivares PR, Rahim F, Riera LS, Villafaina S, Yano Y, Hay SI, Lim SS, Mokdad AH, Naghavi M, Murray CJL. The global burden of falls: global, regional and national estimates of morbidity and mortality from the Global Burden of Disease Study 2017. Inj Prev. 2020 Oct;26(Supp 1):i3-i11. doi: 10.1136/injuryprev-2019-043286. Epub 2020 Jan 15. PMID: 31941758; PMCID: PMC7571347.

26 Tuttle CSL, Thang LAN, Maier AB. Markers of inflammation and their association with muscle strength and mass: A systematic review and meta-analysis. Ageing Res Rev. 2020 Dec;64:101185. doi: 10.1016/j.arr.2020.101185. Epub 2020 Sep 26. PMID: 32992047.

27 Bhattacharya, I., et al. (2016). Association of Muscular Strength and Incidence of Type 2 Diabetes. J Am Coll Cardiol, 68(8), 804-805. doi: 10.1016/j.jacc.2016.06.005

28 Reinders, I., et al. (2021). Associations between skeletal muscle mass, inflammatory markers and mortality in older adults. J Cachexia Sarcopenia Muscle, 12(2), 311-319. doi: 10.1002/jcsm.12697

29 Hadi, F., et al. (2019). The role of skeletal muscle in cardiovascular health and disease. Curr Opin Cardiol, 34(4), 401-407. doi: 10.1097/HCO.0000000000000637

30 Tyrovolas, Stefanos et al. "Skeletal muscle mass in relation to 10 year cardiovascular disease incidence among middle aged and older adults: the ATTICA study." *Journal of epidemiology and community health* vol. 74,1 (2020): 26-31. doi:10.1136/jech-2019-212268

31 Naro, A., Milardi, D., Russo, M., Terranova, C., Rizzo, V., Cacciola, A., ... &

Calabrò, R. S. (2017). What do we know about the influence of the muscular system on brain plasticity and cognitive functions? A narrative review. European Journal of Physical and Rehabilitation Medicine, 53(6), 843-853.

32 Carro, E., Trejo, J. L., Busiguina, S., & Torres-Aleman, I. (2001). Circulating insulin-like growth factor I mediates the protective effects of physical exercise against brain insults of different etiology and anatomy. Journal of Neuroscience, 21(15), 5678-5684.

HEALTHY TRAINING

33 Knuiman, P., Hopman, M.T.E. & Mensink, M. Glycogen availability and skeletal muscle adaptations with endurance and resistance exercise. Nutr Metab (Lond) 12, 59 (2015). https://doi.org/10.1186/s12986-015-0055-9

34 Boyle JP, Thompson TJ, Gregg EW, Barker LE, Williamson DF. Projection of the year 2050 burden of diabetes in the US adult population: dynamic modeling of incidence, mortality, and prediabetes prevalence. *Popul Health Metr.* 2010;8:29. Published 2010 Oct 22. doi:10.1186/1478-7954-8-29

35 Coon, P J et al. "Role of body fat distribution in the decline in insulin sensitivity and glucose tolerance with age." *The Journal of clinical endocrinology and metabolism* vol. 75,4 (1992): 1125-32. doi:10.1210/jcem.75.4.1400882

36 *Slow Recovery after Running? New Research Shows Why and What to Do about It.* https://today.appstate.edu/2015/11/30/david-nieman-2. Accessed 22 Mar. 2023.

37 Wewege, M.A., Desai, I., Honey, C. *et al.* The Effect of Resistance Training in Healthy Adults on Body Fat Percentage, Fat Mass and Visceral Fat: A Systematic Review and Meta-Analysis. *Sports Med* 52, 287–300 (2022).

38 Vechetti IJ Jr, Peck BD, Wen Y, Walton RG, Valentino TR, Alimov AP, Dungan CM, Van Pelt DW, von Walden F, Alkner B, Peterson CA, McCarthy JJ. Mechanical overload-induced muscle-derived extracellular vesicles promote adipose tissue lipolysis. FASEB J. 2021 Jun;35(6):e21644. doi: 10.1096/fj.202100242R. PMID: 34033143; PMCID: PMC8607211.

39 Hackney, K. J., Engels, H. J., & Gretebeck, R. J. (2008). Resting energy expenditure and delayed-onset muscle soreness after full-body resistance training with an eccentric concentration. Journal of Strength and Conditioning Research, 22(5), 1602-1609. doi: 10.1519/JSC.0b013e31818222c5

40 Schuenke, M. D., Mikat, R. P., & McBride, J. M. (2002). Effect of an acute period of resistance exercise on excess post-exercise oxygen consumption: Implications for body mass management. European Journal of Applied

Physiology, 86(5), 411-417. doi: 10.1007/s00421-001-0568-y

41 Godfrey, R. J., Madgwick, Z., & Whyte, G. P. (2003). The exercise-induced growth hormone response in athletes. Sports Medicine, 33(8), 599-613.

42 Kraemer, W. J., & Ratamess, N. A. (2005). Hormonal responses and adaptations to resistance exercise and training. Sports Medicine, 35(4), 339-361.

43 Kraemer, W. J., Hakkinen, K., Newton, R. U., Nindl, B. C., Volek, J. S., McCormick, M., ... & Fleck, S. J. (1998). Effects of heavy-resistance training on hormonal response patterns in younger vs. older men. Journal of Applied Physiology, 85(3), 982-992.

44 Häkkinen, K., Pakarinen, A., Alen, M., Kauhanen, H., & Komi, P. V. (1988). Neuromuscular and hormonal adaptations in athletes to strength training in two years. Journal of Applied Physiology, 65(6), 2406-2412.

45 Cornelissen, V. A., & Smart, N. A. (2013). Exercise training for blood pressure: A systematic review and meta-analysis. Journal of the American Heart Association, 2(1), e004473. doi: 10.1161/JAHA.112.004473

46 Ruiz, J. R., Sui, X., Lobelo, F., Morrow, J. R., Jackson, A. W., Sjöström, M., & Blair, S. N. (2008). Association between muscular strength and mortality in men: Prospective cohort study. BMJ, 337, a439. doi: 10.1136/bmj.a439

47 Fiatarone, M. A., Marks, E. C., Ryan, N. D., Meredith, C. N., Lipsitz, L. A., & Evans, W. J. (1990). High-intensity strength training in nonagenarians: Effects on skeletal muscle. JAMA, 263(22), 3029-3034. doi:10.1001/jama.1990.03440220053029

48 Osteoporosis Fast Facts. Bone Health and Osteoporosis Foundation. PDF. https://www.bonehealthandosteoporosis.org/wp-content/uploads/2015/1 2/Osteoporosis-Fast-Facts.pdf

49 Ye, Q., Wang, B., & Mao, J. (2020). The pathogenesis and treatment of the 'Cytokine Storm' in COVID-19. Journal of Infection, 80(6), 607-613. doi:10.1016/j.jinf.2020.03.037

50 Tregoning, J. S., Brown, E. S., Cheeseman, H. M., Flight, K. E., Higham, S. L., Lemm, N. M., ... & Shattock, R. J. (2021). Vaccines for COVID-19. Clinical & Experimental Immunology, 204(2), 162-192. doi:10.1111/cei.13562

51 Gabay, C., & Kushner, I. (1999). Acute-phase proteins and other systemic responses to inflammation. New England Journal of Medicine, 340(6), 448-454. doi:10.1056/NEJM199902113400607

52 Pedersen, B. K., & Febbraio, M. A. (2008). Muscle as an endocrine organ:

Focus on muscle-derived interleukin-6. Physiological Reviews, 88(4), 1379-1406. doi:10.1152/physrev.90100.2007

53 Pedersen, B. K., & Febbraio, M. A. (2012). Muscles, exercise and obesity: Skeletal muscle as a secretory organ. Nature Reviews Endocrinology, 8(8), 457-465. doi:10.1038/nrendo.2012.49

54 Fyfe, J. J., Bishop, D. J., & Stepto, N. K. (2014). Interference between concurrent resistance and endurance exercise: Molecular bases and the role of individual training variables. Sports Medicine, 44(6), 743-762. doi:10.1007/s40279-014-0162-1

55 Cotman, C. W., & Berchtold, N. C. (2002). Exercise: A behavioral intervention to enhance brain health and plasticity. Trends in Neurosciences, 25(6), 295-301. doi:10.1016/s0166-2236(02)02143-4

56 Matthews, V. B., Aström, M. B., Chan, M. H., Bruce, C. R., Krabbe, K. S., Prelovsek, O., ... & Febbraio, M. A. (2009). Brain-derived neurotrophic factor is produced by skeletal muscle cells in response to contraction and enhances fat oxidation via activation of AMP-activated protein kinase. Diabetologia, 52(7), 1409-1418. doi:10.1007/s00125-009-1364-1

57 Pedersen, B. K., & Febbraio, M. A. (2012). Muscles, exercise and obesity: Skeletal muscle as a secretory organ. Nature Reviews Endocrinology, 8(8), 457-465. doi:10.1038/nrendo.2012.49

58 Knaepen, K., Goekint, M., Heyman, E. M., & Meeusen, R. (2010). Neuroplasticity: Exercise-induced response of peripheral brain-derived neurotrophic factor. Sports Medicine, 40(9), 765-801. doi:10.2165/11534530-000000000-0000

59 McPherron, A. C., Lawler, A. M., & Lee, S. J. (1997). Regulation of skeletal muscle mass in mice by a new TGF-beta superfamily member. Nature, 387(6628), 83-90. doi:10.1038/387083a0

60 Willoughby, D. S. (2004). Effects of heavy resistance training on myostatin mRNA and protein expression. Medicine & Science in Sports & Exercise, 36(4), 574-582. doi:10.1249/01.mss.0000121944.19275.e0

61 Fiems, L. O. (2012). Double muscling in cattle: Genes, husbandry, carcasses and meat. Animals, 2(3), 472-506. doi:10.3390/ani2030472

62 Alway, S. E., Morissette, M. R., & Perrault, T. M. (1999). Myostatin, a negative regulator of muscle mass: Implications for muscle degenerative diseases. Current Genomics, 3(2), 135-156. doi:10.2174/1389202023350467

63 Fernandez-Sola, J. (2010). Muscular adaptations to resistance exercise

in the elderly. Journal of Aging and Physical Activity, 18(4), 441-448. doi:10.1123/japa.18.4.441

64 Lee, S. J., & McPherron, A. C. (2001). Regulation of myostatin activity and muscle growth. Proceedings of the National Academy of Sciences, 98(16), 9306-9311. doi:10.1073/pnas.151270098

65 Miura, T., Kishioka, Y., Wakamatsu, J., Hattori, A., Hennebry, A., Berry, C. J., ... & Sharma, M. (2006). Decorin binds myostatin and modulates its activity to muscle cells. Biochemical and Biophysical Research Communications, 340(2), 675-680. doi:10.1016/j.bbrc.2005.12.060

66 Amthor, H., Otto, A., Vulin, A., Rochat, A., Dumonceaux, J., Garcia, L., ... & Schwander, M. (2009). Muscle hypertrophy driven by myostatin blockade does not require stem/precursor-cell activity. Proceedings of the National Academy of Sciences, 106(18), 7479-7484. doi:10.1073/pnas.0811129106

67 Iozzo, R. V., Buraschi, S., Genua, M., Xu, S. Q., Solomides, C. C., Peiper, S. C., ... & Gomella, L. G. (2011). Decorin antagonizes IGF receptor I (IGF-IR) function by interfering with IGF-IR activity and attenuating downstream signaling. Journal of Biological Chemistry, 286(40), 34712-34721. doi:10.1074/jbc.M111.262766

68 Gilson, H., Schakman, O., Kalista, S., Lause, P., Tsuchida, K., & Thissen, J. P. (2009). Follistatin induces muscle hypertrophy through satellite cell proliferation and inhibition of both myostatin and activin. American Journal of Physiology-Endocrinology and Metabolism, 297(1), E157-E164. doi:10.1152/ajpendo.00193.2009

69 Garry, G. A., Antony, M. L., Garry, D. J., & Kumar, A. (2016). Follistatin therapeutic enhances the quality of life in the mdx mouse. Neuromuscular Disorders, 26(9), 624-629. doi:10.1016/j.nmd.2016.06.449

70 Moore, J. B., & June, C. H. (2020). Cytokine release syndrome in severe COVID-19. Science, 368(6490), 473-474. doi:10.1126/science.abb8925

71 Pedersen, B. K., & Febbraio, M. A. (2008). Muscle as an endocrine organ: focus on muscle-derived interleukin-6. Physiological Reviews, 88(4), 1379-1406. doi:10.1152/physrev.90100.2007

72 Fischer, C. P. (2006). Interleukin-6 in acute exercise and training: what is the biological relevance? Exercise Immunology Review, 12, 6-33. PMID: 17201070

73 Steensberg, A., Fischer, C. P., Keller, C., Moller, K., & Pedersen, B. K. (2003). IL-6 enhances plasma IL-1ra, IL-10, and cortisol in humans. American

Journal of Physiology-Endocrinology and Metabolism, 285(2), E433-E437. doi:10.1152/ajpendo.00074.2003

74 Carey, A. L., Steinberg, G. R., Macaulay, S. L., Thomas, W. G., Holmes, A. G., Ramm, G., ... & Febbraio, M. A. (2006). Interleukin-6 increases insulin-stimulated glucose disposal in humans and glucose uptake and fatty acid oxidation in vitro via AMP-activated protein kinase. Diabetes, 55(10), 2688-2697. doi:10.2337/db05-1404

75 Serrano, A. L., Baeza-Raja, B., Perdiguero, E., Jardí, M., & Muñoz-Cánoves, P. (2008). Interleukin-6 is an essential regulator of satellite cell-mediated skeletal muscle hypertrophy. Cell Metabolism, 7(1), 33-44. doi:10.1016/j.cmet.2007.11.011

76 Frost, R. A., & Lang, C. H. (2003). Protein kinase B/Akt: a nexus of growth factor and cytokine signaling in determining muscle mass. Journal of Applied Physiology, 95(1), 272-278. doi:10.1152/japplphysiol.00089.2003

77 Peake, J. M., Della Gatta, P., & Cameron-Smith, D. (2010). Aging and its effects on inflammation in skeletal muscle at rest and following exercise-induced muscle injury. American Journal of Physiology-Regulatory, Integrative and Comparative Physiology, 298(6), R1485-R1495. doi:10.1152/ajpregu.00467.2009

78 Bostrom, P., Wu, J., Jedrychowski, M. P., Korde, A., Ye, L., Lo, J. C., ... & Spiegelman, B. M. (2012). A PGC1-α-dependent myokine that drives brown-fat-like development of white fat and thermogenesis. Nature, 481(7382), 463-468. doi:10.1038/nature10777

79 Colaianni, G., Cuscito, C., & Colucci, S. (2015). Irisin Enhances Osteoblast Differentiation In Vitro. International Journal of Endocrinology, 2015, 902186. doi:10.1155/2015/902186

80 Moreno-Navarrete, J. M., Ortega, F., Serrano, M., Guerra, E., Pardo, G., Tinahones, F., ... & Fernandez-Real, J. M. (2013). Irisin is expressed and produced by human muscle and adipose tissue in association with obesity and insulin resistance. The Journal of Clinical Endocrinology & Metabolism, 98(4), E769-E778. doi:10.1210/jc.2012-2749

81 Wrann, C. D., White, J. P., Salogiannnis, J., Laznik-Bogoslavski, D., Wu, J., Ma, D., ... & Spiegelman, B. M. (2013). Exercise induces hippocampal BDNF through a PGC-1α/FNDC5 pathway. Cell Metabolism, 18(5), 649-659. doi:10.1016/j.cmet.2013.09.008

82 Gannon, N. P., Vaughan, R. A., & Garcia-Smith, R. (2015). Effects of the exercise-inducible myokine irisin on malignant and non-malignant breast

epithelial cell behavior in vitro. International Journal of Cancer, 136(4), E197-E202. doi:10.1002/ijc.29142

83 Vaughan, R. A., Gannon, N. P., & Barberena, M. A. (2014). Characterization of the metabolic effects of irisin on skeletal muscle in vitro. Diabetes, Obesity and Metabolism, 16(8), 711-718. doi:10.1111/dom.12268

84 Rao, R. R., Long, J. Z., White, J. P., Svensson, K. J., Lou, J., Lokurkar, I., ... & Spiegelman, B. M. (2014). Meteorin-like is a hormone that regulates immune-adipose interactions to increase beige fat thermogenesis. Cell, 157(6), 1279-1291. doi:10.1016/j.cell.2014.03.065

85 Bae, J. Y., Woo, J., Kang, S., Shin, K. O., & Jang, K. S. (2018). Exercise-induced myokines can explain the importance of physical activity in the elderly: an overview. Aging Clinical and Experimental Research, 30(7), 729-736. doi:10.1007/s40520-018-0953-5

86 Church, D. D., Hoffman, J. R., Mangine, G. T., Jajtner, A. R., Townsend, J. R., Beyer, K. S., ... & Stout, J. R. (2016). Comparison of high-intensity vs. high-volume resistance training on the BDNF response to exercise. Journal of Applied Physiology, 121(1), 123-128.

87 Wrann, C. D., White, J. P., Salogiannnis, J., Laznik-Bogoslavski, D., Wu, J., Ma, D., ... & Spiegelman, B. M. (2013). Exercise induces hippocampal BDNF through a PGC-1α/FNDC5 pathway. Cell Metabolism, 18(5), 649-659.

88 Nielsen, A. R., & Pedersen, B. K. (2007). The biological roles of exercise-induced cytokines: IL-6, IL-8, and IL-15. Applied Physiology, Nutrition, and Metabolism, 32(5), 833-839.

89 Rao, R. R., Long, J. Z., White, J. P., Svensson, K. J., Lou, J., Lokurkar, I., ... & Spiegelman, B. M. (2014). Meteorin-like is a hormone that regulates immune-adipose interactions to increase beige fat thermogenesis. Cell, 157(6), 1279-1291.

90 Gordon, B. R., McDowell, C. P., Hallgren, M., Meyer, J. D., Lyons, M., & Herring, M. P. (2018). Association of efficacy of resistance exercise training with depressive symptoms: Meta-analysis and meta-regression analysis of randomized clinical trials. JAMA Psychiatry, 75(6), 566-576.

91 Strickland, J. C., & Smith, M. A. (2014). The anxiolytic effects of resistance exercise. Frontiers in Psychology, 5, 753.

92 Gordon, B. R., McDowell, C. P., Lyons, M., & Herring, M. P. (2017). The effects of resistance exercise training on anxiety: A meta-analysis and meta-regression analysis of randomized controlled trials. Sports Medicine, 47(12), 2521-2532.

93 Marquez, C. M. S., Vanaudenaerde, B., Troosters, T., & Wenderoth, N. (2015). High-intensity interval training evokes larger serum BDNF levels compared with intense continuous exercise. Journal of Applied Physiology, 119(12), 1363-1373.

WHAT IS STRENGTH TRAINING?

94 Ratamess, N. A., Alvar, B. A., Evetoch, T. K., Housh, T. J., Kibler, W. B., Kraemer, W. J., & Triplett, N. T. (2009). Progression models in resistance training for healthy adults. Medicine & Science in Sports & Exercise, 41(3), 687-708.

95 Moritani, T., & deVries, H. A. (1979). Neural factors versus hypertrophy in the time course of muscle strength gain. American Journal of Physical Medicine, 58(3), 115-130.

96 Schoenfeld, B. J., Grgic, J., & Krieger, J. (2019). How many times per week should a muscle be trained to maximize muscle hypertrophy? A systematic review and meta-analysis of studies examining the effects of resistance training frequency. Journal of Sports Sciences, 37(11), 1286-1295.

97 Morton, R. W., Oikawa, S. Y., Wavell, C. G., Mazara, N., McGlory, C., Quadri-latero, J., ... & Phillips, S. M. (2016). Neither load nor systemic hormones determine resistance training-mediated hypertrophy or strength gains in resistance-trained young men. Journal of Applied Physiology, 121(1), 129-138.

98 Rhea, M. R., Alvar, B. A., Burkett, L. N., & Ball, S. D. (2003). A meta-analysis to determine the dose response for strength development. Medicine & Science in Sports & Exercise, 35(3), 456-464.

99 Kraemer, W. J., & Ratamess, N. A. (2004). Fundamentals of resistance training: progression and exercise prescription. Medicine & Science in Sports & Exercise, 36(4), 674-688.

100 Sale, D. G. (1988). Neural adaptation to resistance training. Medicine and science in sports and exercise, 20(5 Suppl), S135-45.

101 Folland, J. P., & Williams, A. G. (2007). The adaptations to strength training: morphological and neurological contributions to increased strength. Sports Medicine, 37(2), 145-168.

102 Fleck, S. J., & Kraemer, W. J. (2014). Designing resistance training programs. Human Kinetics.

103 Schoenfeld, B. J., Ogborn, D., & Krieger, J. W. (2017). Dose-response relationship between weekly resistance training volume and increases in

muscle mass: A systematic review and meta-analysis. Journal of Sports Sciences, 35(11), 1073-1082.

GETTING STARTED

104 Aagaard, P., Simonsen, E. B., Andersen, J. L., Magnusson, P., & Dyhre-Poulsen, P. (2002). Increased rate of force development and neural drive of human skeletal muscle following resistance training. Journal of applied physiology, 93(4), 1318-1326.

105 Moritani, T., & deVries, H. A. (1979). Neural factors versus hypertrophy in the time course of muscle strength gain. American Journal of Physical Medicine, 58(3), 115-130.

HIGH-PROTEIN

106 Wolfe, R. R., Cifelli, A. M., Kostas, G., & Kim, I. Y. (2017). Optimizing Protein Intake in Adults: Interpretation and Application of the Recommended Dietary Allowance Compared with the Acceptable Macronutrient Distribution Range. Advances in Nutrition, 8(2), 266-275.

107 Wu, Guoyao. "Dietary protein intake and human health." Food & function vol. 7,3 (2016): 1251-65. doi:10.1039/c5fo01530h

108 Stuart M.PhillipsS.M. Phillips. Dietary protein for athletes: from requirements to metabolic advantage. Applied Physiology, Nutrition, and Metabolism. 31(6): 647-654. https://doi.org/10.1139/h06-035

109 Krok-Schoen, J.L., Archdeacon Price, A., Luo, M. et al. Low Dietary Protein Intakes and Associated Dietary Patterns and Functional Limitations in an Aging Population: A NHANES Analysis. J Nutr Health Aging 23, 338–347 (2019). https://doi.org/10.1007/s12603-019-1174-1

110 U.S. Department of Agriculture, Agricultural Research Service. (2016). Nutrient Intakes from Food and Beverages: Mean Amounts Consumed per Individual, by Gender and Age. Retrieved from **https://www.ars.usda.gov/ARSUserFiles/80400530/pdf/1516/Table_1_NIN_GEN_15.pdf**

111 Brouns, F. (2018). Overweight and diabetes prevention: is a low-carbohydrate-high-fat diet recommendable? European Journal of Nutrition, 57(4), 1301-1312. doi:10.1007/s00394-018-1636-y

112 Paoli, A. (2014). Ketogenic diet for obesity: friend or foe? International Journal of Environmental Research and Public Health, 11(2), 2092-2107. doi:10.3390/ijerph110202092

113 Schwingshackl, L., & Hoffmann, G. (2013). Low-fat versus low-

carbohydrate diets: a systematic review and meta-analysis. Nutrition Journal, 12(1), 146. doi:10.1186/1475-2891-12-146

114 Institute of Medicine (US) Panel on Macronutrients. (2005). Dietary Reference Intakes for Energy, Carbohydrate, Fiber, Fat, Fatty Acids, Cholesterol, Protein, and Amino Acids. National Academies Press. Retrieved from **https://www.ncbi.nlm.nih.gov/books/NBK56068/**

115 Phillips, S. M., & Van Loon, L. J. (2011). Dietary protein for athletes: from requirements to optimum adaptation. Journal of Sports Sciences, 29(Suppl 1), S29–S38. doi:10.1080/02640414.2011.619204

HIGH-PROTEIN HEALTH BENEFITS

116 Luppino, F. S., de Wit, L. M., Bouvy, P. F., Stijnen, T., Cuijpers, P., Penninx, B. W., & Zitman, F. G. (2010). Overweight, obesity, and depression: a systematic review and meta-analysis of longitudinal studies. Archives of general psychiatry, 67(3), 220-229.

117 Markus, C. R., Olivier, B., de Haan, E. H., & Wheal, H. V. (2002). Protein-rich breakfasts improve linear and verbal reasoning in schoolchildren. The American journal of clinical nutrition, 75(4), 767-773.

118 Boelsma, E., Brink, E. J., Stafleu, A., Hendriks, H. F., & Meijer, G. W. (2007). Protein supplementation improves alertness and cognitive function in long-term care residents with low serum albumin. Journal of the American Medical Directors Association, 8(5), 322-327.

119 Urska Dobersek, Kelsey Teel, Sydney Altmeyer, Joshua Adkins, Gabrielle Wy, Jackson Peak. (2021) Meat and mental health: A meta-analysis of meat consumption, depression, and anxiety. *Critical Reviews in Food Science and Nutrition* 0:0, pages 1-18.

120 Thomas P Wycherley, Lisa J Moran, Peter M Clifton, Manny Noakes, Grant D Brinkworth, Effects of energy-restricted high-protein, low-fat compared with standard-protein, low-fat diets: a meta-analysis of randomized controlled trials, The American Journal of Clinical Nutrition, Volume 96, Issue 6, December 2012, Pages 1281–1298, https://doi.org/10.3945/ajcn.11 2.044321

121 Soenen S, Westerterp-Plantenga MS. Changes in body fat percentage during body weight stable conditions of increased daily protein intake vs. control. Physiol Behav. 2010 Dec 2;101(5):635-8. doi: 10.1016/j.physbeh.2010.09.014. Epub 2010 Sep 29. PMID: 20887742.

122 Aller, E., Larsen, T., Claus, H. et al. Weight loss maintenance in overweight

subjects on ad libitum diets with high or low protein content and glycemic index: the DIOGENES trial 12-month results. Int J Obes 38, 1511–1517 (2014). https://doi.org/10.1038/ijo.2014.52

123 Alexandra M Johnstone, Graham W Horgan, Sandra D Murison, David M Bremner, Gerald E Lobley, Effects of a high-protein ketogenic diet on hunger, appetite, and weight loss in obese men feeding ad libitum, The American Journal of Clinical Nutrition, Volume 87, Issue 1, January 2008, Pages 44–55, https://doi.org/10.1093/ajcn/87.1.44

124 Thomas L. Halton & Frank B. Hu (2004) The Effects of High Protein Diets on Thermogenesis, Satiety and Weight Loss: A Critical Review, Journal of the American College of Nutrition, 23:5, 373-385, DOI: 10.1080/07315724.2004.10719381

125 Marion Journel, Catherine Chaumontet, Nicolas Darcel, Gilles Fromentin, Daniel Tomé, Brain Responses to High-Protein Diets, Advances in Nutrition, Volume 3, Issue 3, May 2012, Pages 322–329, https://doi.org/10.3945/an.112.002071

126 Tischmann L, Drummen M, Gatta-Cherifi B, Raben A, Fogelholm M, Hartmann B, Holst JJ, Matias I, Cota D, Mensink RP, Joris PJ, Westerterp-Plantenga MS, Adam TC. Effects of a High-Protein/Moderate-Carbohydrate Diet on Appetite, Gut Peptides, and Endocannabinoids—A Preview Study. Nutrients. 2019; 11(10):2269. https://doi.org/10.3390/nu11102269

127 Leidy HJ, Lepping RJ, Savage CR, Harris CT. Neural responses to visual food stimuli after a normal vs. higher protein breakfast in breakfast-skipping teens: a pilot fMRI study. Obesity (Silver Spring). 2011 Oct;19(10):2019-25. doi: 10.1038/oby.2011.108. Epub 2011 May 5. PMID: 21546927; PMCID: PMC4034051.

128 Westerterp, K.R. Diet induced thermogenesis. Nutr Metab (Lond) 1, 5 (2004). https://doi.org/10.1186/1743-7075-1-5

129 Larsen TM, Dalskov SM, van Baak M, Jebb SA, Papadaki A, Pfeiffer AF, Martinez JA, Handjieva-Darlenska T, Kunešová M, Pihlsgård M, Stender S, Holst C, Saris WH, Astrup A; Diet, Obesity, and Genes (Diogenes) Project. Diets with high or low protein content and glycemic index for weight-loss maintenance. N Engl J Med. 2010 Nov 25;363(22):2102-13. doi: 10.1056/NEJMoa1007137. PMID: 21105792; PMCID: PMC3359496.

130 Wycherley, Thomas P et al. "A high-protein diet with resistance exercise training improves weight loss and body composition in overweight and obese patients with type 2 diabetes." Diabetes care vol. 33,5 (2010): 969-76.

doi:10.2337/dc09-1974

131 Jay J. Cao, LuAnn K. Johnson, Janet R. Hunt, A Diet High in Meat Protein and Potential Renal Acid Load Increases Fractional Calcium Absorption and Urinary Calcium Excretion without Affecting Markers of Bone Resorption or Formation in Postmenopausal Women, The Journal of Nutrition, Volume 141, Issue 3, March 2011, Pages 391–397, https://doi.org/10.3945/jn.110.129361

132 J E Kerstetter, D M Caseria, M E Mitnick, A F Ellison, L F Gay, T A Liskov, T O Carpenter, K L Insogna, Increased circulating concentrations of parathyroid hormone in healthy, young women consuming a protein-restricted diet, The American Journal of Clinical Nutrition, Volume 66, Issue 5, November 1997, Pages 1188–1196, https://doi.org/10.1093/ajcn/66.5.1188

133 Jane E. Kerstetter, Kimberly O. O'Brien, Donna M. Caseria, Diane E. Wall, Karl L. Insogna, The Impact of Dietary Protein on Calcium Absorption and Kinetic Measures of Bone Turnover in Women, The Journal of Clinical Endocrinology & Metabolism, Volume 90, Issue 1, 1 January 2005, Pages 26–31, https://doi.org/10.1210/jc.2004-0179

134 Ronald G Munger, James R Cerhan, Brian C-H Chiu, Prospective study of dietary protein intake and risk of hip fracture in postmenopausal women, The American Journal of Clinical Nutrition, Volume 69, Issue 1, January 1999, Pages 147–152, https://doi.org/10.1093/ajcn/69.1.147

135 McAuley, K.A., Hopkins, C.M., Smith, K.J. et al. Comparison of high-fat and high-protein diets with a high-carbohydrate diet in insulin-resistant obese women. Diabetologia 48, 8–16 (2005). https://doi.org/10.1007/s00125-004-1603-4

136 Helms, Eric R., Caryn Zinn, David S. Rowlands, Ruth Naidoo, and John Cronin. "High-Protein, Low-Fat, Short-Term Diet Results in Less Stress and Fatigue Than Moderate-Protein, Moderate-Fat Diet During Weight Loss in Male Weightlifters: A Pilot Study". International Journal of Sport Nutrition and Exercise Metabolism 25.2 (2015): 163-170. < https://doi.org/10.1123/ijsnem.2014-0056>. Web. 14 Feb. 2023.

137 Campbell, W. W., Johnson, C. A., McCabe, G. P., Carnell, N. S., & Pasiakos, S. M. (2018). Dietary protein requirements of younger and older adults. The American Journal of Clinical Nutrition, 108(1), 70-79.

138 Calder, P. C. (2017). Feeding the immune system. Proceedings of the Nutrition Society, 76(3), 237- 242.

139 Deley, G., Leduc-Gaudet, J. P., Reynaud, O., Gouspillou, G., Sgarioto, N., Labrecque, G., ... & Morais, J. A. (2017). Increased protein requirements in elderly people: new data and retrospective reassessments. Frontiers in Nutrition, 4, 17.

140 Leidy, H. J., Gwin, J. A., Roenfeldt, C. A., Zino, A. Z., & Shafer, R. S. (2018). Evaluating the intervention-based evidence surrounding the causal role of breakfast on markers of weight management, with specific focus on breakfast composition and size. Advances in Nutrition, 9(6), 717-725.

141 Iddir M, Brito A, Dingeo G, Fernandez Del Campo SS, Samouda H, La Frano MR, Bohn T. Strengthening the Immune System and Reducing Inflammation and Oxidative Stress through Diet and Nutrition: Considerations during the COVID-19 Crisis. Nutrients. 2020; 12(6):1562. https://doi.org/1 0.3390/nu12061562

142 He J, et al. Effects of dietary protein intervention on blood pressure: a meta-analysis of randomized controlled trials. Am J Clin Nutr. 2011;94(3):780-788. doi:10.3945/ajcn.111.018148

143 Karianna FM Teunissen-Beekman, Janneke Dopheide, Johanna M Geleijnse, Stephan JL Bakker, Elizabeth J Brink, Peter W de Leeuw, Marleen A van Baak, Protein supplementation lowers blood pressure in overweight adults: effect of dietary proteins on blood pressure (PROPRES), a randomized trial, The American Journal of Clinical Nutrition, Volume 95, Issue 4, April 2012, Pages 966–971, https://doi.org/10.3945/ajcn.111.029116

144 Wang X, et al. Effect of a moderate high-protein diet on lipid metabolism, glycemic control, insulin sensitivity, and body composition in type 2 diabetes: a randomized controlled trial. J Am Coll Cardiol. 2011;58(3):268-277. doi:10.1016/j.jacc.2011.03.047

COMMON QUESTIONS & CONCERNS

145 Antonio, J., Peacock, C.A., Ellerbroek, A. *et al.* The effects of consuming a high protein diet (4.4 g/kg/d) on body composition in resistance-trained individuals. *J Int Soc Sports Nutr* 11, 19 (2014). https://doi.org/10.1186/1550-2783-11-19

146 Antonio, J., Ellerbroek, A., Silver, T. *et al.* A high protein diet (3.4 g/kg/d) combined with a heavy resistance training program improves body composition in healthy trained men and women – a follow-up investigation. *J Int Soc Sports Nutr* 12, 39 (2015). https://doi.org/10.1186/s12970-015-0100-0

HOW TO GET STARTED

147 Alpana P. Shukla, Radu G. Iliescu, Catherine E. Thomas, Louis J. Aronne; Food Order Has a Significant Impact on Postprandial Glucose and Insulin Levels. *Diabetes Care* 1 July 2015; 38 (7): e98–e99. https://doi.org/10.2337/dc15-0429

SLEEP, MUSCLE, AND HEALTH

148 Di H, Guo Y, Daghlas I, et al. Evaluation of Sleep Habits and Disturbances Among US Adults, 2017-2020. *JAMA Netw Open.* 2022;5(11):e2240788. doi:10.1001/jamanetworkopen.2022.40788

149 Van Cauter, E., Leproult, R., & Plat, L. (2000). Age-related changes in slow wave sleep and REM sleep and relationship with growth hormone and cortisol levels in healthy men. JAMA, 284(7), 861-868.

150 Peyreigne, C., Bouix, D., Micallef, J. P., Mercier, J., Bringer, J., Préfaut, C., & Brun, J. F. (1998). Exercise-induced growth hormone secretion and hemorheology during exercise in elite athletes. Clinical Hemorheology and Microcirculation, 18(2-3), 245-254.

151 Leproult, R., & Van Cauter, E. (2011). Effect of 1 week of sleep restriction on testosterone levels in young healthy men. JAMA, 305(21), 2173-2174.

152 Afonso, V. M., Lui, M. A., & Gooley, J. J. (2018). Sleep and muscle recovery: Endocrinological and molecular basis for a new and promising hypothesis. Medical Hypotheses, 119, 74-79.

153 Trommelen, J., & Van Loon, L. J. (2016). Pre-sleep protein ingestion to improve the skeletal muscle adaptive response to exercise training. Nutrients, 8(12), 763.

154 Besedovsky, L., Lange, T., & Born, J. (2012). Sleep and immune function. Pflügers Archiv-European Journal of Physiology, 463(1), 121-137.

155 Cappuccio, F. P., Cooper, D., D'Elia, L., Strazzullo, P., & Miller, M. A. (2011). Sleep duration predicts cardiovascular outcomes: a systematic review and meta-analysis of prospective studies. European Heart Journal, 32(12), 1484-1492.

156 Drager, L. F., Togeiro, S. M., Polotsky, V. Y., & Lorenzi-Filho, G. (2011). Obstructive sleep apnea: a cardiometabolic risk in obesity and the metabolic syndrome. Journal of the American College of Cardiology, 62(7), 569-576.

157 Laugsand, L. E., Strand, L. B., Platou, C., Vatten, L. J., & Janszky, I. (2014). Insomnia and the risk of incident heart failure: a population study. European Heart Journal, 35(21), 1382-1393.

158 Van Cauter, E., & Knutson, K. L. (2008). Sleep and the epidemic of obesity in children and adults. European Journal of Endocrinology, 159(Supplement 1), S59-S66.

159 Spiegel, K., Leproult, R., & Van Cauter, E. (1999). Impact of sleep debt on metabolic and endocrine function. The Lancet, 354(9188), 1435-1439.

160 Knutson, K. L., Ryden, A. M., Mander, B. A., & Van Cauter, E. (2006). Role of sleep duration and quality in the risk and severity of type 2 diabetes mellitus. Archives of Internal Medicine, 166(16), 1768-1774.

161 Buxton, O. M., Pavlova, M., Reid, E. W., Wang, W., Simonson, D. C., & Adler, G. K. (2010). Sleep restriction for 1 week reduces insulin sensitivity in healthy men. Diabetes, 59(9), 2126-2133.

162 Kahn, S. E., Hull, R. L., & Utzschneider, K. M. (2006). Mechanisms linking obesity to insulin resistance and type 2 diabetes. Nature, 444(7121), 840-846.

163 Cappuccio, F. P., Taggart, F. M., Kandala, N. B., Currie, A., Peile, E., Stranges, S., & Miller, M. A. (2008). Meta-analysis of short sleep duration and obesity in children and adults. Sleep, 31(5), 619-626.

164 Spiegel, K., Tasali, E., Penev, P., & Van Cauter, E. (2004). Brief communication: Sleep curtailment in healthy young men is associated with decreased leptin levels, elevated ghrelin levels, and increased hunger and appetite. Annals of internal medicine, 141(11), 846-850.

165 Müller, T. D., Nogueiras, R., Andermann, M. L., Andrews, Z. B., Anker, S. D., Argente, J., ... & Leibel, R. L. (2011). Ghrelin. Molecular Metabolism, 30(10), 939-962.

166 Taheri, S., Lin, L., Austin, D., Young, T., & Mignot, E. (2004). Short sleep duration is associated with reduced leptin, elevated ghrelin, and increased body mass index. PLoS medicine, 1(3), e62.

167 Knutson, K. L., Spiegel, K., Penev, P., & Van Cauter, E. (2007). The metabolic consequences of sleep deprivation. Sleep medicine reviews, 11(3), 163-178.

168 Van Cauter, E., Spiegel, K., Tasali, E., & Leproult, R. (2008). Metabolic consequences of sleep and sleep loss. Sleep medicine, 9, S23-S28.

169 Koren, D., Dumin, M., & Gozal, D. (2011). Role of sleep quality in the metabolic syndrome. Diabetes, Metabolic Syndrome and Obesity: Targets and Therapy, 4, 261-271.

170 Baron, K. G., Reid, K. J., & Zee, P. C. (2013). Exercise to improve sleep in insomnia: exploration of the bidirectional effects. Journal of clinical sleep

medicine, 9(8), 819-824.

171 Valdes, A. M., Walter, J., Segal, E., & Spector, T. D. (2018). Role of the gut microbiota in nutrition and health. BMJ, 361, k2179. **https://doi.org/10.1136/bmj.k2179**

172 Cryan, J. F., & Dinan, T. G. (2012). Mind-altering microorganisms: the impact of the gut microbiota on brain and behaviour. Nature Reviews Neuroscience, 13(10), 701–712. **https://doi.org/10.1038/nrn3346**

173 Benedict, C., Vogel, H., Jonas, W., Woting, A., Blaut, M., Schürmann, A., & Cedernaes, J. (2016). Gut microbiota and glucometabolic alterations in response to recurrent partial sleep deprivation in normal-weight young individuals. Molecular Metabolism, 5(12), 1175-1186. **https://doi.org/10.1016/j.molmet.2016.10.003**

174 Rogers, G. B., Keating, D. J., Young, R. L., Wong, M. L., Licinio, J., & Wesselingh, S. (2016). From gut dysbiosis to altered brain function and mental illness: mechanisms and pathways. Molecular Psychiatry, 21(6), 738–748. **https://doi.org/10.1038/mp.2016.50**

175 Konturek, P. C., Brzozowski, T., & Konturek, S. J. (2011). Stress and the gut: pathophysiology, clinical consequences, diagnostic approach and treatment options. Journal of Physiology and Pharmacology, 62(6), 591-599. Retrieved from **http://www.jpp.krakow.pl/journal/archive/12_11/pdf/591_12_11_article.pdf**

176 Smith, R. P., Easson, C., Lyle, S. M., Kapoor, R., Donnelly, C. P., Davidson, E. J., Parikh, E., Lopez, J. V., & Tartar, J. L. (2019). Gut microbiome diversity is associated with sleep physiology in humans. PLoS ONE, 14(10), e0222394. **https://doi.org/10.1371/journal.pone.0222394**

177 Walker, M. P. (2017). Why We Sleep: Unlocking the Power of Sleep and Dreams. Scribner.

178 Diekelmann, S., & Born, J. (2010). The memory function of sleep. Nature Reviews Neuroscience, 11(2), 114–126. **https://doi.org/10.1038/nrn2762**

179 Baglioni, C., Battagliese, G., Feige, B., Spiegelhalder, K., Nissen, C., Voderholzer, U., Lombardo, C., & Riemann, D. (2011). Insomnia as a predictor of depression: a meta-analytic evaluation of longitudinal epidemiological studies. Journal of Affective Disorders, 135(1-3), 10-19. **https://doi.org/10.1016/j.jad.2011.01.011**

180 Alvaro, P. K., Roberts, R. M., & Harris, J. K. (2013). A Systematic Review Assessing Bidirectionality between Sleep Disturbances, Anxiety, and Depression. Sleep, 36(7), 1059–1068. **https://doi.org/10.5665/sleep.2810**

181 Staner, L. (2003). Sleep and anxiety disorders. Dialogues in Clinical Neuroscience, 5(3), 249-258. Retrieved from **https://www.ncbi.nlm.nih.gov/pmc/articles/PMC3181635/**

182 Killgore, W. D. (2010). Effects of sleep deprivation on cognition. Progress in Brain Research, 185, 105-129. **https://doi.org/10.1016/B978-0-444-53702-7.00007-5**

183 Durmer, J. S., & Dinges, D. F. (2005). Neurocognitive Consequences of Sleep Deprivation. Seminars in Neurology, 25(1), 117–129. **https://doi.org/10.1055/s-2005-867080**

184 Diekelmann, S., & Born, J. (2010). The memory function of sleep. Nature Reviews Neuroscience, 11(2), 114–126. **https://doi.org/10.1038/nrn2762**

185 Akerstedt, T. (2006). Psychosocial stress and impaired sleep. Scandinavian Journal of Work, Environment & Health, 32(6), 493-501. **https://doi.org/10.5271/sjweh.1054**

186 Germain, A. (2013). Sleep disturbances as the hallmark of PTSD: where are we now? The American Journal of Psychiatry, 170(4), 372-382. **https://doi.org/10.1176/appi.ajp.2012.12040432**

187 Kobayashi, I., Boarts, J. M., & Delahanty, D. L. (2007). Polysomnographically measured sleep abnormalities in PTSD: A meta-analytic review. Psychophysiology, 44(4), 660-669. **https://doi.org/10.1111/j.1469-8986.2007.00559.x**

188 Yoo, S. S., Gujar, N., Hu, P., Jolesz, F. A., & Walker, M. P. (2007). The human emotional brain without sleep—a prefrontal amygdala disconnect. Current Biology, 17(20), R877-R878. **https://doi.org/10.1016/j.cub.2007.08.007**

189 Finan, P. H., Goodin, B. R., & Smith, M. T. (2013). The association of sleep and pain: An update and a path forward. The Journal of Pain, 14(12), 1539-1552. **https://doi.org/10.1016/j.jpain.2013.08.007**

190 Krause, A. J., Prather, A. A., Wager, T. D., Lindquist, M. A., & Walker, M. P. (2019). The pain of sleep loss: A brain characterization in humans. The Journal of Neuroscience, 39(12), 2291-2300. **https://doi.org/10.1523/JNEUROSCI.2408-18.2018**

191 Besedovsky, L., Lange, T., & Haack, M. (2019). The sleep-immune crosstalk in health and disease. Physiological Reviews, 99(3), 1325-1380. **https://doi.org/10.1152/physrev.00010.2018**

192 Roehrs, T., Hyde, M., Blaisdell, B., Greenwald, M., & Roth, T. (2006). Sleep loss and REM sleep loss are hyperalgesic. Sleep, 29(2), 145-151. **https://doi.org/10.1093/sleep/29.2.145**

193 Davison, S. L., & Bell, R. J. (2006). Androgen levels in adult females: changes with age, menopause, and oophorectomy. The Journal of Clinical Endocrinology & Metabolism, 91(7), 2841-2847.

194 Luboshitzky, R., Zabari, Z., Shen-Orr, Z., Herer, P., & Lavie, P. (2001). Disruption of the nocturnal testosterone rhythm by sleep fragmentation in normal men. The Journal of Clinical Endocrinology & Metabolism, 86(3), 1134-1139.

195 Hamilton, L. D., & Meston, C. M. (2011). Chronic stress and sexual function in women. Journal of Sexual Medicine, 8(10), 2777-2783.

196 Hirotsu, C., Tufik, S., & Andersen, M. L. (2015). Interactions between sleep, stress, and metabolism: From physiological to pathological conditions. Sleep Science, 8(3), 143-152.

197 Baglioni, C., Battagliese, G., Feige, B., Spiegelhalder, K., Nissen, C., Voder-holzer, U., Lombardo, C., & Riemann, D. (2011). Insomnia as a predictor of depression: A meta-analytic evaluation of longitudinal epidemiological studies. Journal of Affective Disorders, 135(1-3), 10-19.

198 Kennedy, S. H., & Rizvi, S. (2009). Sexual dysfunction, depression, and the impact of antidepressants. Journal of Clinical Psychopharmacology, 29(2), 157-164.

GETTING ENOUGH

199 Hastings, M., O'Neill, J. S., & Maywood, E. S. (2007). Circadian clocks: regulators of endocrine and metabolic rhythms. Journal of Endocrinology, 195(2), 187-198.

200 Foster, R. G., & Kreitzman, L. (2014). The rhythms of life: what your body clock means to you! Experimental Physiology, 99(4), 599-606.

201 Potter, G. D., Skene, D. J., Arendt, J., Cade, J. E., Grant, P. J., & Hardie, L. J. (2016). Circadian rhythm and sleep disruption: causes, metabolic consequences, and countermeasures. Endocrine Reviews, 37(6), 584-608.

202 Janszky, I., & Ljung, R. (2008). Shifts to and from daylight saving time and incidence of myocardial infarction. New England Journal of Medicine, 359(18), 1966-1968.

203 Carskadon, M. A., & Dement, W. C. (2011). Monitoring and staging human sleep. In Principles and Practice of Sleep Medicine (pp. 16-26). Elsevier.

204 Meerlo, P., Sgoifo, A., & Suchecki, D. (2008). Restricted and disrupted sleep: effects on autonomic function, neuroendocrine stress systems and stress responsivity. Sleep Medicine Reviews, 12(3), 197-210.

205 Silber, M. H., Ancoli-Israel, S., Bonnet, M. H., Chokroverty, S., Grigg-Damberger, M. M., Hirshkowitz, M., ... & Kushida, C. A. (2007). The visual scoring of sleep in adults. Journal of Clinical Sleep Medicine, 3(2), 121-131.

206 Van Cauter, E., Plat, L., & Copinschi, G. (1998). Interrelations between sleep and the somatotropic axis. Sleep, 21(6), 553-566.

207 Walker, M. P. (2009). The role of sleep in cognition and emotion. Annals of the New York Academy of Sciences, 1156(1), 168-197.

208 Aeschbach, D., Borbély, A. A., & Dijk, D. J. (1997). Dynamics of EEG spindle frequency activity during extended sleep in humans: relationship to slow-wave activity and time of day. Brain Research, 748(1-2), 131-136.

209 Xie, L., Kang, H., Xu, Q., Chen, M. J., Liao, Y., Thiyagarajan, M., ... & Nedergaard, M. (2013). Sleep drives metabolite clearance from the adult brain. Science, 342(6156), 373-377.

210 Andersen, M. L., & Tufik, S. (2008). The effects of testosterone on sleep and sleep-disordered breathing in men: its bidirectional interaction with erectile function. Sleep Medicine Reviews, 12(5), 365-379.

211 Van Cauter, E., Plat, L., & Copinschi, G. (1998). Interrelations between sleep and the somatotropic axis. Sleep, 21(6), 553-566.

212 Samuels, M. H. (2008). Effects of variations in physiological cortisol levels on thyrotropin secretion in subjects with adrenal insufficiency: a clinical research center study. The Journal of Clinical Endocrinology & Metabolism, 93(3), 929-934.

213 Brambilla, D. J., Matsumoto, A. M., Araujo, A. B., & McKinlay, J. B. (2009). The effect of diurnal variation on clinical measurement of serum testosterone and other sex hormone levels in men. The Journal of Clinical Endocrinology & Metabolism, 94(3), 907-913.

214 Zisapel, N. (2001). Melatonin-dopamine interactions: from basic neurochemistry to a clinical setting. Cellular and Molecular Neurobiology, 21(6), 605-616.

215 Spiegel, K., Leproult, R., & Van Cauter, E. (1999). Impact of sleep debt on metabolic and endocrine function. The Lancet, 354(9188), 1435-1439.

216 Buckley, T. M., & Schatzberg, A. F. (2005). On the interactions of the hypothalamic-pituitary-adrenal (HPA) axis and sleep: normal HPA axis activity and circadian rhythm, exemplary sleep disorders. Journal of Clinical Endocrinology & Metabolism, 90(5), 3106-3114.

SLEEP HYGIENE

217 Ebrahim et al. "Alcohol and sleep I: effects on normal sleep." Alcoholism, Clinical and Experimental Research, vol. 37, no.4, 2013, pp. 539-549.

218 Tolstrup et al. "Alcohol consumption and sleep in middle-aged men and women." Addiction, vol. 105, no. 2, 2010, pp. 277-278.

219 Roehrs et al. "Alcohol and sleep II: effects on daytime sleepiness, performance, and mood." Alcoholism, Clinical and Experimental Research, vol. 37, no.4, 2013, pp. 598-604.

220 Roenneberg, T., Allebrandt, K. V., Merrow, M., & Vetter, C. (2012). Social jetlag and obesity. Current Biology, 22(10), 939-943.

221 Okamoto-Mizuno, K., & Mizuno, K. (2012). Effects of thermal environment on sleep and circadian rhythm. Journal of Physiological Anthropology, 31(1), 14.

222 Askenasy JJ, Goldstein R. Does a subtropical climate imply a seasonal rhythm in REM sleep? Sleep. 1995 Dec;18(10):895-900. doi: 10.1093/sleep/18.10.895. PMID: 8746398.

223 Chang, A. M., Aeschbach, D., Duffy, J. F., & Czeisler, C. A. (2015). Evening use of light-emitting eReaders negatively affects sleep, circadian timing, and next-morning alertness. Proceedings of the National Academy of Sciences, 112(4), 1232-1237.

224 Black, D. S., O'Reilly, G. A., Olmstead, R., Breen, E. C., & Irwin, M. R. (2015). Mindfulness meditation and improvement in sleep quality and daytime impairment among older adults with sleep disturbances: A randomized clinical trial. JAMA Internal Medicine, 175(4), 494-501.

225 Slutsky, I., Abumaria, N., Wu, L. J., Huang, C., Zhang, L., Li, B., ... & Tonegawa, S. (2010). Enhancement of learning and memory by elevating brain magnesium. Neuron, 65(2), 165-177. **https://doi.org/10.1016/j.neuron.2010.01.003**

226 Abbasi, B., Kimiagar, M., Sadeghniiat, K., Shirazi, M. M., Hedayati, M., & Rashidkhani, B. (2012). The effect of magnesium supplementation on primary insomnia in elderly: A double-blind placebo-controlled clinical trial. Journal of Research in Medical Sciences: The Official Journal of Isfahan University of Medical Sciences, 17(12), 1161-1169. **https://www.ncbi.nlm.nih.gov/pmc/articles/PMC3703169/**

227 Nielsen, F. H., Johnson, L. K., & Zeng, H. (2010). Magnesium supplementation improves indicators of low magnesium status and inflammatory stress in adults older than 51 years with poor quality sleep. Magnesium Research, 23(4), 158-168. **https://doi.org/10.1684/mrh.2010.0220**

228 Koulivand, P. H., Ghadiri, M. K., & Gorji, A. (2013). Lavender and the Nervous System. Evidence-Based Complementary and Alternative Medicine, 2013, 1-10.

229 Hwang, E., & Shin, S. (2015). The effects of aromatherapy on sleep improvement: A systematic literature review and meta-analysis. Journal of Alternative and Complementary Medicine, 21(2), 61-68.

230 Koulivand, P. H., Ghadiri, M. K., & Gorji, A. (2013). Lavender and the Nervous System. Evidence-Based Complementary and Alternative Medicine, 2013, 1-10.

231 Chang, Y. Y., Lin, C. L., & Chang, C. Y. (2018). The Effects of Aromatherapy Massage on Sleep Quality of Nurses on Monthly Rotating Night Shifts. Evidence-Based Complementary and Alternative Medicine, 2018, 1-6.

232 Seol, G. H., Shim, H. S., Kim, P. J., Moon, H. K., Lee, K. H., Shim, I., Suh, S. H., & Min, S. S. (2010). Antidepressant-like effect of Salvia sclarea is explained by modulation of dopamine activities in rats. Journal of Ethnopharmacology, 130(1), 187-190.

233 Watanabe, E., Kuchta, K., Kimura, M., Rauwald, H. W., Kamei, T., & Imanishi, J. (2015). Effects of bergamot (Citrus bergamia (Risso) Wright & Arn.) essential oil aromatherapy on mood states, parasympathetic nervous system activity, and salivary cortisol levels in 41 healthy females. Complementary Therapies in Medicine, 23(1), 58-62.

234 Bent, S., Padula, A., Moore, D., Patterson, M., & Mehling, W. (2006). Valerian for sleep: A systematic review and meta-analysis. The American Journal of Medicine, 119(12), 1005-1012.

235 Garrison, R., & Chambliss, W. G. (2006). Effect of a proprietary Magnolia and Phellodendron extract on weight management: A pilot, double-blind, placebo-controlled clinical trial. Alternative Therapies in Health and Medicine, 12(1), 50-54.

236 Talbott, S. M., Talbott, J. A., Pugh, M., & Alt, A. (2013). Effect of Magnolia officinalis and Phellodendron amurense (Relora®) on cortisol and psychological mood state in moderately stressed subjects. Journal of the International Society of Sports Nutrition, 10(1), 37.

237 Kalman, D. S., Feldman, S., Feldman, R., Schwartz, H. I., Krieger, D. R., & Garrison, R. (2008). Effect of a proprietary Magnolia and Phellodendron extract on stress levels in healthy women: A pilot, double-blind, placebo-controlled clinical trial. Nutrition Journal, 7(1), 11.

238 Mody, I. (2001). Distinguishing between GABA(A) receptors responsible for tonic and phasic conductances. Neurochemical Research, 26(8-9), 907-913.

239 Abdou, A. M., Higashiguchi, S., Horie, K., Kim, M., Hatta, H., & Yokogoshi, H. (2006). Relaxation and immunity enhancement effects of γ-Aminobutyric acid (GABA) administration in humans. BioFactors, 26(3), 201-208.

240 Yamatsu, A., Yamashita, Y., Pandharipande, T., Maru, I., & Kim, M. (2015). Effect of oral γ-aminobutyric acid (GABA) administration on sleep and its absorption in humans. Food Science and Biotechnology, 24(2), 585-589.

241 Birdsall, T. C. (1998). 5-Hydroxytryptophan: A clinically-effective serotonin precursor. Alternative Medicine Review, 3(4), 271-280.

242 Arendt, J. (2005). Melatonin: Characteristics, concerns, and prospects. Journal of Biological Rhythms, 20(4), 291-303.

243 Shell, W., Bullias, D., Charuvastra, E., May, L. A., & Silver, D. S. (2010). A randomized, placebo-controlled trial of an amino acid preparation on timing and quality of sleep. American Journal of Therapeutics, 17(2), 133-139.

244 Kimura, K., Ozeki, M., Juneja, L. R., & Ohira, H. (2007). L-Theanine reduces psychological and physiological stress responses. Biological Psychology, 74(1), 39-45.

245 Hidese, S., Ogawa, S., Ota, M., Ishida, I., & Yasukawa, Z. (2019). Effects of L-Theanine administration on stress-related symptoms and cognitive functions in healthy adults: A randomized controlled trial. Nutrients, 11(10), 2362.

246 Nathan, P. J., Lu, K., Gray, M., & Oliver, C. (2006). The neuropharmacology of L-theanine (N-ethyl-L-glutamine): a possible neuroprotective and cognitive enhancing agent. Journal of Herbal Pharmacotherapy, 6(2), 21-30.

247 Lyon, M. R., Kapoor, M. P., & Juneja, L. R. (2011). The effects of L-theanine (Suntheanine®) on objective sleep quality in boys with attention deficit hyperactivity disorder (ADHD): a randomized, double-blind, placebo-controlled clinical trial. Alternative Medicine Review, 16(4), 348-354.

248 Ota, M., Wakabayashi, C., Sato, N., Hori, H., Hattori, K., Hori, H., ... & Kunugi, H. (2015). Effect of L-theanine on glutamatergic function in patients with schizophrenia. Acta Neuropsychiatrica, 27(5), 291-296.

249 Arendt, J. (2005). Melatonin: characteristics, concerns, and prospects. Journal of Biological Rhythms, 20(4), 291-303.

250 Cajochen, C., Kräuchi, K., & Wirz-Justice, A. (2003). Role of melatonin in the regulation of human circadian rhythms and sleep. Journal of Neuroendocrinology, 15(4), 432-437.

251 Brainard, G. C., Hanifin, J. P., Greeson, J. M., Byrne, B., Glickman, G., Gerner, E., & Rollag, M. D. (2001). Action spectrum for melatonin regulation in humans: evidence for a novel circadian photoreceptor. Journal of Neuroscience, 21(16), 6405-6412.

252 Auld, F., Maschauer, E. L., Morrison, I., Skene, D. J., & Riha, R. L. (2017). Evidence for the efficacy of melatonin in the treatment of primary adult sleep disorders. Sleep Medicine Reviews, 34, 10-22.

253 Zhdanova, I. V., Wurtman, R. J., Morabito, C., Piotrovska, V. R., & Lynch, H. J. (1995). Effects of low oral doses of melatonin, given 2-4 hours before habitual bedtime, on sleep in normal young humans. Sleep, 18(5), 333-339.

254 Jin, X., von Gall, C., Pieschl, R. L., Gribkoff, V. K., Stehle, J. H., Reppert, S. M., & Weaver, D. R. (2003). Targeted disruption of the mouse Mel(1b) melatonin receptor. Molecular and Cellular Biology, 23(3), 1054-1060.

255 Miles, A., & Philbrick, D. R. S. (1988). Melatonin and psychiatry. Biological Psychiatry, 23(4), 405-425.

256 Rossignol, D. A., & Frye, R. E. (2011). Melatonin in autism spectrum disorders: a systematic review and meta-analysis. Developmental Medicine & Child Neurology, 53(9), 783-792.

257 Wade, A. G., Ford, I., Crawford, G., McMahon, A. D., Nir, T., Laudon, M., & Zisapel, N. (2010). Efficacy of prolonged release melatonin in insomnia patients aged 55-80 years: quality of sleep and next-day alertness outcomes. Current Medical Research and Opinion, 26(10), 2419-2431.

DEALING WITH OBSTACLES

258 Breen, L., & Phillips, S. M. (2011). Skeletal muscle protein metabolism in the elderly: Interventions to counteract the 'anabolic resistance' of ageing. Nutrients, 3(10), orus 441-458.

259 Kumar, V., Selby, A., Rankin, D., Patel, R., Atherton, P., Hildebrandt, W., ... & Rennie, M. J. (2009). Age-related differences in the dose-response relationship of muscle protein synthesis to resistance exercise in young and old men. The Journal of Physiology, 587(1), 211-217.

BEYOND THE 3 PILLARS

260 Huang HY, Caballero B, Chang S, et al. The efficacy and safety of mul-

tivitamin and mineral supplement use to prevent cancer and chronic disease in adults: a systematic review for a National Institutes of Health state-of-the-science conference. Ann Intern Med. 2006;145(5):372-385. doi:10.7326/0003-4819-145-5-200609050-00135

261 Bailey RL, Fulgoni VL 3rd, Keast DR, et al. Examination of vitamin intakes among US adults by dietary supplement use. J Acad Nutr Diet. 2012;112(5):657-663.e4. doi:10.1016/j.jand.2011.12.002

262 Ames BN. Prevention of mutation, cancer, and other age-associated diseases by optimizing micronutrient intake. J Nucleic Acids. 2010;2010:Article ID 725071. doi:10.4061/2010/725071

263 Miller PE, Van Elswyk M, Alexander DD. Long-chain omega-3 fatty acids eicosapentaenoic acid and docosahexaenoic acid and blood pressure: a meta-analysis of randomized controlled trials. Am J Hypertens. 2014;27(7):885-896. doi: 10.1093/ajh/hpu024.

264 Lee YH, Bae SC, Song GG. Omega-3 polyunsaturated fatty acids and the treatment of rheumatoid arthritis: a meta-analysis. Arch Med Res. 2012;43(5):356-362. doi: 10.1016/j.arcmed.2012.06.011.

265 Grosso G, Galvano F, Marventano S, et al. Omega-3 fatty acids and depression: scientific evidence and biological mechanisms. Oxid Med Cell Longev. 2014;2014:313570. doi: 10.1155/2014/313570.

266 Bhargava R, Kumar P, Kumar M, Mehra N, Mishra A. A randomized controlled trial of omega-3 fatty acids in dry eye syndrome. Int J Ophthalmol. 2013;6(6):811-816. doi: 10.3980/j.issn.2222-3959.2013.06.14.

267 Brouwer IA, Geleijnse JM, Klaasen VM, et al. n-3 fatty acids, ventricular arrhythmia-related events, and fatal myocardial infarction in postmyocardial infarction patients with diabetes. Diabetes Care. 2013;36(7):2015-2022. doi: 10.2337/dc12-2219.

268 Castiglioni S, Cazzaniga A, Albisetti W, Maier JA. Magnesium and osteoporosis: current state of knowledge and future research directions. Nutrients. 2013;5(8):3022-3033. doi: 10.3390/nu5083022.

269 Hruby A, Meigs JB, O'Donnell CJ, Jacques PF, McKeown NM. Higher magnesium intake reduces risk of impaired glucose and insulin metabolism, and progression from prediabetes to diabetes in middle-aged Americans. Diabetes Care. 2013;36(3):594-599. doi: 10.2337/dc12-0685.

270 Abbasi B, Kimiagar M, Sadeghniiat K, Shirazi MM, Hedayati M, Rashidkhani B. The effect of magnesium supplementation on primary insomnia in

elderly: a double-blind placebo-controlled clinical trial. J Res Med Sci. 2012;17(12):1161-1169.

271 Mauskop A, Varughese J. Why all migraine patients should be treated with magnesium. J Neural Transm (Vienna). 2012;119(5):575-579. doi: 10.1007/s00702-012-0790-2.

272 Boyle NB, Lawton C, Dye L. The effects of magnesium supplementation on subjective anxiety and stress-a systematic review. Nutrients. 2017;9(5):429. doi: 10.3390/nu9050429.

273 Mansbach, JM, & Ginde, AA. (2009). Vitamin D for prevention of viral upper respiratory infections.

274 Cannell, JJ, Vieth, R, Umhau, JC, Holick, MF, Grant, WB, Madronich, S, & Garland, CF. (2006). Epidemic influenza and vitamin D. Epidemiol Infect, 134(6), 1129-1140.

275 Holick, MF. (2011). Vitamin D: A D-lightful solution for health. J Investig Med, 59(6), 872-880.

276 Urashima, M, Segawa, T, Okazaki, M, Kurihara, M, & Wada, Y. (2010). Randomized trial of vitamin D supplementation to prevent seasonal influenza A in schoolchildren. Am J Clin Nutr, 91(5), 1255-1260.

277 Pittas, AG, Dawson-Hughes, B, Li, T, Van Dam, RM, Willett, WC, & Manson, JE. (2007). Vitamin D and calcium intake in relation to type 2 diabetes in women. Diabetes Care, 30(3), 650-656.

278 Holick, MF. (2011). Vitamin D: A D-lightful solution for health. J Investig Med, 59(6), 872-880.

279 Keim, NL, Garcia, DO, Garcia-Marcos, PW, Lutes, AC, & Symonds, ME. (2020). Vitamin D status during pregnancy and child cognitive and behavioural development: A systematic review. Matern Child Nutr, 16(4), e12948.

280 Didari, T, Mozaffari, S, Nikfar, S, & Abdollahi, M. (2014). Effectiveness of probiotics in irritable bowel syndrome: Updated systematic review with meta-analysis. World Journal of Gastroenterology, 20(34), 14853-14867.

281 Sharma, S, Vijayendra, SVN, & Rao, LJM. (2018). Health benefits of fermented foods: Microbiota and beyond. Current Opinion in Biotechnology, 49, 129-134.

282 Wallace, CJK, & Milev, R. (2017). The effects of probiotics on depressive symptoms in humans: A systematic review. Annals of General Psychiatry, 16(1), 14.

283 Suarez F, Levitt M, Adshead J, Barkin J. Pancreatic supplements reduce symptomatic response of healthy subjects to a high fat meal. Dig Dis Sci. 1999;44(7):1317-1321.

284 Moolchandani K, Saigal S, Kamboj AK, et al. Efficacy of enzyme supplementation in malnourished children with diarrhea. J Pediatr Gastroenterol Nutr. 2018;67(2):e26-e30.

285 Brien S, Lewith G, Walker A, Hicks SM, Middleton D. Bromelain as a treatment for osteoarthritis: a review of clinical studies. Evid Based Complement Alternat Med. 2004;1(3):251-257.

286 Miller PC, Bailey SP, Barnes ME, Derr SJ, Hall EE. The effects of protease supplementation on skeletal muscle function and DOMS following downhill running. J Sports Sci. 2004;22(4):365-372.

287 Biswas, A., et al. (2015). Sedentary time and its association with risk for disease incidence, mortality, and hospitalization in adults: a systematic review and meta-analysis. Annals of Internal Medicine, 162(2), 123-132.

288 Mekary, R.A., et al. (2012). Sitting time and mortality from all causes, cardiovascular disease, and cancer. Medicine and Science in Sports and Exercise, 44(5), 998-1005.

289 Owen, N., et al. (2010). Sedentary behavior: emerging evidence for a new health risk. Mayo Clinic Proceedings, 85(12), 1138-1141.

290 Dempsey, P.C., et al. (2016). Interrupting prolonged sitting in type 2 diabetes: nocturnal persistence of improved glycaemic control. Diabetologia, 59(3), 550-558.

291 Yates, T., et al. (2015). Stand up for your health: Is it time to rethink the physical activity paradigm? Diabetes Research and Clinical Practice, 110(2), 195-197.

292 Bakrania, K., et al. (2018). Associations of objectively measured sedentary behaviour and physical activity with markers of cardiometabolic health. Diabetologia, 61(11), 2500-2510.

293 Benatti FB, Ried-Larsen M. The effects of breaking up prolonged sitting time: a review of experimental studies. Med Sci Sports Exerc. 2015;47(10):2053-61. doi: 10.1249/MSS.0000000000000654. PMID: 26378968.

294 Healy GN, Dunstan DW, Salmon J, et al. Breaks in sedentary time: beneficial associations with metabolic risk. Diabetes Care. 2008;31(4):661-666. doi: 10.2337/dc07-2046. PMID: 18252904.

295 Bailey DP, Locke CD. Breaking up prolonged sitting with light-intensity walking improves postprandial glycemia, but breaking up sitting with standing does not. J Sci Med Sport. 2015;18(3):294-298. doi: 10.1016/j.jsams.2014.03.008. PMID: 24768683.

296 Peddie MC, Bone JL, Rehrer NJ, Skeaff CM, Gray AR, Perry TL. Breaking prolonged sitting reduces postprandial glycemia in healthy, normal-weight adults: a randomized crossover trial. Am J Clin Nutr. 2013;98(2):358-366. doi: 10.3945/ajcn.112.051763. PMID: 23803881.

297 Pulsford RM, Blackwell J, Hillsdon M, et al. Objectively measured sedentary time and its association with markers of cardiometabolic health and fitness among cardiac patients. Int J Cardiol. 2014;177(2):536-541. doi: 10.1016/j.ijcard.2014.09.142. PMID: 25444480.

298 Wilmot EG, Edwardson CL, Achana FA, et al. Sedentary time in adults and the association with diabetes, cardiovascular disease and death: systematic review and meta-analysis. Diabetologia. 2012;55(11):2895-2905. doi: 10.1007/s00125-012-2677-z. PMID: 22890825.

299 Chau JY, Grunseit A, Midthjell K, et al. Sedentary behaviour and risk of mortality from all-causes and cardiometabolic diseases in adults: evidence from the HUNT3 population cohort. Br J Sports Med. 2015;49(11):737-742. doi: 10.1136/bjsports-2014-093524. PMID: 25899294.

300 Ohkawara K, Cornier MA, Kohrt WM, Melanson EL. Effects of increased meal frequency on fat oxidation and perceived hunger. *Obesity (Silver Spring)*. 2013;21(2):336-343. doi:10.1002/oby.20032

301 Kahleova, Hana et al. "Meal Frequency and Timing Are Associated with Changes in Body Mass Index in Adventist Health Study 2." *The Journal of nutrition* vol. 147,9 (2017): 1722-1728. doi:10.3945/jn.116.244749

302 Lopez-Minguez J, Gómez-Abellán P, Garaulet M. Timing of Breakfast, Lunch, and Dinner. Effects on Obesity and Metabolic Risk. *Nutrients*. 2019;11(11):2624. Published 2019 Nov 1. doi:10.3390/nu11112624

CONCLUDING THOUGHTS

303 Christakis, N. A., & Fowler, J. H. (2007). The spread of obesity in a large social network over 32 years. New England journal of medicine, 357(4), 370-379.

304 University of Pennsylvania. (2016). Exercise more effective with a partner. ScienceDaily. Retrieved from
www.sciencedaily.com/releases/2016/05/160518141423.htm

305 Holt-Lunstad, J., Smith, T. B., & Layton, J. B. (2010). Social relationships and mortality risk: a meta-analytic review. PLoS medicine, 7(7), e1000316.